"*Noting Left to Give*" is a refreshing departure from the dense academic literature on burnout. As someone in the healthcare field who provides training on topics such as burnout and compassion fatigue, I appreciate the book's down-to-earth approach. Dr. Obianyor's relatable stories help readers identify and express their burnout experiences, creating a connection that many academic resources lack. What sets this book apart is its commitment to practical solutions. It doesn't just outline symptoms but offers actionable tips to confront and manage burnout. In a world where burnout is prevalent, *'Nothing Left to Give'* serves as a valuable companion, providing a roadmap to healing and resilience. Dr. Obianyor's work is a must-read for anyone seeking a pragmatic guide to understand and overcome burnout.

—*Anonymous Reviewer*

Praise for 'Nothing Left to Give'

I have known Dr. Florence *(aka Dr. Flo)* for many years and more closely in the past 2 years. I have witnessed Dr. Flo's passion for mental health demonstrated in a very deep and genuine way. She usually tells me that her involvement in mental health care does not diminish her energy rather it energizes her to do more. I have definitely seen that displayed. Dr. Flo's fervent interest in mental health is not merely an academic or professional pursuit, it is a deeply personal and empathetic quest. She does not write this book as a detached observer from the ivory tower but as a compassionate guide. She has crafted this book as someone who has traversed the labyrinth of their own emotions and emerged with insights that shimmer with authenticity.

This book offers a beacon of solace for those navigating the labyrinth of their own emotions, struggles and challenges. May this book serve as a lantern in the darkness, illuminating your path towards knowing that you are not alone in your struggles, understanding the steps it takes to start your healing and help you discover the profound resilience that resides in you.

— *Dr. Yemisi Adewale*

"Dr. Florence Obianyor's *'Nothing Left to Give'* compassionately navigates the complex landscape of energy depletion, offering insightful guidance and practical strategies for individuals struggling with exhaustion. A must-read for holistic wellness."

—*Engr. Christopher Ifejika (MNSE, COREN)*

This is a book that every clinician, especially the patient facing ones need to read. The issue of burnout is a common negative experience and the consequence of it can be both career and life redefining. Showing vulnerability is not a very common attribute of doctors! Writing a book like this is quite commendable, because Dr. Obianyor decided to speak and write on something quite taboo amongst us. Hopefully many of us will be more intuitive and seek help when needed to save our family attendant stress and to be able to continue to give great care to our patients.

—*Dr Daniel Olu*

Florence Obianyor, a medical Doctor, takes a deep vulnerable dive to share her burnout journey. She tackles various burdens in our society. Especially workplace takes a large toll on us. Where striving for excellence erodes emotionally, physically, and mentally. Professionals like engineers, business analysts, and accountants all have their own perspectives and how they came to realize that they were also at burnout's door. She addresses this issue by showing not only the difficulties, but proffers solutions.

This is not a normal textbook on burnout, but a real deep dive into the very crux of the matter. By dropping problems at the seabed and picking up remedies you can swim safely to shore. Well done Dr. Flo.

—*Margaret Isabel, Houston, TX*

The Preface for this wonderfully riveting book was the first item that caught my attention. The author stated that it was her dream to write a book. Just to write a book, this book – *'Nothing Left to Give'*— is a great feat!

The book bravely details her journey through life, a journey that deliciously spices the intent of the book – identifying *'Burnout'* and managing it. The biographical mix resonated deeply with me, and I am certain that this mix will appeal to persons who have had the experience of settling, working in new and unfamiliar environments and conditions.

I have experienced burnout, and seeing how one who encountered and defeated it is inspiring for me. I enjoyed reading this book and I highly recommend it too!

—*Engr Samson Obianyor, MNSE*

NOTHING LEFT TO GIVE

IDENTIFY AND OVERCOME BURNOUT
TO GET YOUR LIFE BACK ON TRACK.

FLORENCE OBIANYOR, MD

Copyright © 2023 by Florence Obianyor

All rights reserved. No part of this publication may be reproduced, stored in a retrieval system or transmitted in any form or by any means electronic, mechanical, photocopying, recording or otherwise without the prior permission of the author.

For permissions and other inquiries, visit drflo.net/contact

All Scripture quotations, unless otherwise indicated, are taken from the Holy Bible, New International Version®, NIV®. Copyright ©1973, 1978, 1984, 2011 by Biblica, Inc.™ Used by permission of Zondervan. All rights reserved worldwide. www.zondervan.com The "NIV" and "New International Version" are trademarks registered in the United States Patent and Trademark Office by Biblica, Inc.™

Cover photography by Samuel Obadero
Book Layout by Toluwanimi Babarinde

ISBN: 978-17-38172-00-9
Printed in Canada

CONTENTS

DEDICATION	IX
PREFACE	XI
INTRODUCTION	XIII
THE SILENT ONSET OF BURNOUT	**1**
Tracing Burnout's Ember	1
Drained: The Vehicle-Battery Analogy	2
Measuring Burnout	5
Meet And Greet With Burnout	6
Culture Creates Burnout	19
THE CULPRIT WITHIN	**19**
System Culture As A Burnout Driver	20
Organizational Culture: Burnout's Ally	22
Perfectionism: The Talent Trap	23
Organizational Culture: Burnout's Playground	27
Carla The Nurse	28
Kai The Business Analyst	31
People-Pleasing To Perishing	35
THE DOMINO EFFECT	**35**
Consequences Of Excessive Stress (Burnout)	38
Angie The Senior Administrative Secretary	40
Curtis And Trish, The Accountants	42
Andrew The Engineer	45
Unveiling Personal Culture: A Deep Dive	46
FINDING YOUR HEALING	**55**
Cultural Crossroads	56
Focusing On Leaders	*64*
Focusing On Clients	*66*
Personal Work-Related Strategies	67
The Wellness-Resilience Factor	75
THE MIRACLE OF GETTING AWAY	**75**
The Practice Of Mindfulness And Meditation	*77*
Self-Awareness, Forgiveness And Self-Compassion	*78*
The Power Of Pause	*80*
The Power Of Sleep	*81*

Sleep Induction: Progressive Muscular Relaxation. 83
The Wisdom Of Wanderlust 83
Fearful Skies 86
Healing Through Fitness *91*

THE BODY'S ABILITY TO HEAL THROUGH FITNESS AND FOOD **91**
Nature's Therapy 92
Summit And Saddle 94
Glide And Grace 95
Building Your Fitness Haven 95
Dancing Like No One's Watching 97
Mind-Body Harmony *97*
Energy Flow 98
Culinary Healing 99
Hydrate To Heal *107*
Buzz And Burnout 107
Substances *108*
Maintaining Peak Physical Health 109
Genetics And Medication Compliance 111
Healing Through Community *117*

THE POWER OF SOCIAL CONNECTIONS **117**
Connect With Your Younger Self 121
Creative Therapies 121
Tapping Into Higher Powers *127*

THE GIFT OF SPIRITUALITY **127**
Recover & Rebuild with Professional Care 135

THE COURAGE TO DO IT DIFFERENTLY **135**
The Role Of Primary Care Providers And Therapists 136
The Role Of Life Coach 140
Role Of Financial Advisors And Accountants 141
Personal And Professional Development 145

RECHARGED AND READY **147**
ACTION PLAN **153**
CONCLUSION **155**
APPENDIX **159**
REFERENCES **161**
GLOSSARY OF TERMS **165**

DEDICATION

This book is dedicated to my parents, who are deceased and have been resting in peace for many years now. They were instrumental in creating the person I have turned out to be: a curious and fearless individual, an advocate for fairness and justice, striving only for the very best there is, and making a positive impact in the lives of those I come into contact with.

I also dedicate this book to my children Anthony, Sean, and Kendra for their love and for challenging what I know to be the best in a way that has made me less of me and more of my Creator, whom I have come to rely on now more than ever before.

My dedication would be incomplete without those who have done life with me in one form or the other. This includes those who were not supportive, for they forced me to look further into myself to discover the real me and the passion I have. It is this reflection that has molded me and refined me. Thank you.

To those who have brought about my dream of being an author, thank you, for without you, my ideas and stories would have remained exactly that: ideas and stories. To put pen to paper is a dream come true not just in terms of self-actualization, but a step in the right direction to help many others at once in conquering barriers impacting their physical, mental, and emotional health.

PREFACE

I have always wanted to write books since childhood. Somehow I stumbled upon journaling at an early age and kept diaries for over thirty years, despite not knowing exactly what stories to either share with the world or what the world itself would care to hear about. My love for learning and improvement is endless! It is this passion that brings me into the world of writing for the betterment of all.

Sir Winston Churchill wrote *'courage is what it takes to stand up and speak; courage is also what it takes to sit down and listen.'* I have a few books in draft form, but chose to start with this book on burnout considering how rampant an issue it is today than ever before. This is based on the literature and my observation that a higher number of my clients are experiencing burnout lately.

Many do not know why they are feeling the way they are until their symptoms are pieced together to arrive at a burnout diagnosis. Hence, there is an urgent need to address it now.

However, before we go into the book, here's a little about me. I graduated from medical school over twenty years ago as a General Practitioner. My sojourn in Canada led to additional training at the University of Calgary; hence I'm certified to practice Family Medicine by the College of Family Physicians of Canada. In 2019, I was appointed as a medical expert at the court of Queensbench. I am also a fellow of the College, with over ten years of practice with a passion for mental health and wellness, seniors care, leadership, research and teaching.

Between 2020-2022, I was medical director at a Senior Living Facility in Alberta, Canada. Also a practice reviewer with the College of Physicians and Surgeons of Alberta, Canada, I am a clinical lecturer at the Cumming School of Medicine, and part-time physician advisor, Diversity, Equity and Inclusion, Wellness and Leadership Development.

My love for learning led to a Master in Public Health degree with merit, at the University of Liverpool (U.K.), Fellowship certificate in Health System Improvement at the School of Public Health, University of Alberta, Canada in 2019, and diploma with merit in Clinical Research from Humber Institute, Toronto, Canada in 2007.

Even after a decade of work as a Family Physician with a practice focused on mental health, my passion for improving people's mental health and wellness remains, and it is time to share my discoveries with as many people as possible.

FLORENCE OBIANYOR, MD

INTRODUCTION

Take a look at the following questions:

- *Are you feeling overwhelmed, bogged down, or emotionally exhausted from the day-to-day as though you have nothing left to give?*
- *Are you an immigrant, professional, senior executive, health care worker, resident doctor, practicing physician, nurse, care aide, accountant, teacher, administrator, student, or perhaps a stay-at-home mom juggling multiple tasks daily, or non-professional whose emotional battery is depleted?*
- *Have you felt you no longer know the person staring back at you in the mirror?*
- *Has your personality changed? Do you sense a feeling of detachment from work and from others? Do you sense a lack of excitement from the job you once loved?*
- *Have you found yourself considering quitting your job or switching careers?*
- *Do you desire to have greater energy and increased sense of fulfilment at work? Do you desire to make fewer errors, and experience better satisfaction and interaction with your patients or clients? Do you desire an improved sense of clarity and purpose?*

If you answered *yes to three or more* of these questions, keep this book by your bedside or take it with you on a trip because it might be the best gift you will ever give to yourself or loved one.

You could be experiencing burnout. I say *could* be burnout, because there are other conditions that mimic burnout like sleep apnea, thyroid dysfunction, chronic fatigue syndrome, or anxiety and depression. My goal is to help you clarify if what you are experiencing is burnout and, more importantly, offer some tips for managing and also preventing it in the long term.

If you have never heard the term, you might be asking *'what in the world is burnout?'*

First coined by Herbert Freudenberger in 1975 to explain the *'excessive demands on energy, strength or resources'*[1], burnout still lives among us. Thomas[2] defined burnout as *'a pathological syndrome causing emotional depletion and maladaptive detachment from prolonged occupational stresses'* whereas World Health Organization defined it as a syndrome arising from chronic stress that has not been successfully managed that consists of three components:

- *Feelings of energy depletion or exhaustion;*
- *Increased mental distance from one's job, or feelings of negativism or cynicism related to one's job; and*
- *Reduced professional efficacy.*[3]

Simply put, burnout is a situation that an individual might experience arising from unattended prolonged stress caused by either working excessively or working in a non-healthy work environment. It is not a medical illness, although it can mimic mental health conditions like anxiety, depression, or chronic fatigue.

One of the reasons I'm writing this book now is that burnout is very real. I call it the *Burnout Beast* that needs to be identified for what it is – an enemy. My enemy, *Your enemy.*

In 2010, I did a review of *Burnout in Family Physicians* as my final year research project, and thirteen years later, it is still on the rise. At that time, I found that more than half of urban family physicians experienced burnout[4]. In the United States, *one in five* physicians experiencing burnout were primary care physicians and sub-specialists.[5] In Europe, about two-thirds of physicians experienced burnout.[6]

Interestingly, my findings then are quite similar to today's statistics with regard to burnout risk factors, consequences, and the coping strategies, with only slight variations. Hence, physician burnout was already a global problem long before the COVID-19 pandemic. *The National Physician Health Survey*, conducted by the Canadian Medical Association in 2021, revealed that approximately *half* of physicians were experiencing burnout, with an equivalent prevalence in anxiety and depression[7].

According to the *Survey on Health Care Workers' Experience During the Pandemic* conducted in 2021, a third of nurses indicated that they had plans to spend less than three years at their current jobs. A little over a third of these nurses were considering retirement; for those nurses, job burnout, mental health and well-being concerns and perceived lack of job satisfaction were the top reasons[8].

The COVID-19 virus infection itself began in Wuhan, China around December 2019, which later became a global issue (a pandemic) by March 2020, a situation possibly heightened by the ease of travel (cross-border travel) and immigration, the advancement in technology with larger plane capacity and more plane flights today than ever before for intercontinental businesses, and more leisurely travels. Though, COVID-19 began as a pandemic that affected people unexpectedly worldwide, three years later, it has become an endemic illness, meaning the infection is expected to occur in communities.

The consequences of the pandemic included the scramble for food items, toilet paper, and baby formula — household supplies that were previously not an issue for those in first world countries, let alone third world countries. The cost of living skyrocketed and hospital capacities were overwhelmed due to increased hospitalizations, loss of health care workers to physical illness and mental health challenges. This elevated the perception of hopelessness which further increased burnout globally. Since the pandemic and its impacts were global, it is safe to assume that the issues seen in North America were not very different from elsewhere.

We are yet to fully recover from that shock and the attendant distress it created. For many health care workers, showing up at work each day meant their risk for contracting the virus was higher; and they were also likely to be sources of the virus to their family members. There was also social disconnection (through policies made by many governments in a bid to control the spread of the virus).

Besides the COVID-19 pandemic, there are many other burnout drivers related to the workplace which will be explored in the coming chapters. I'm confident that regardless of what these drivers are, there is hope.

The truth is that burnout is not limited to professions like medicine and nursing; it occurs in the oil and gas industry, education, – in short, wherever people work. And for the burnout veterans, you might wonder, why read yet another book on burnout? In my humble view, this book provides a holistic perspective that has not yet been fully explored.

Given my background as a family doctor with mental health and wellness practice, the comprehensive approach offered in this book might be the true game changer. This approach incorporates some storytelling based on my personal experiences of burnout, and those of clients from various professional backgrounds, thereby increasing the possibility of connecting more easily with the topic than one would otherwise. This means that regardless of where in the stress or burnout cycle you find yourself, you can take a more proactive approach in preventing burnout, or at minimum add a couple more tools to your current arsenal for managing burnout.

One thing is certain — no one ever achieved a different result doing things the way they did it before. In this book, I will show you how to identify and manage burnout, and when to seek professional help. I will also share additional tips for thriving at the workplace.

Burnout has lived amongst us for too long. It is time for real change. To do nothing or to take a less than comprehensive approach is to foster the burnout culture.

Are you willing to have an open mind and consider trying things differently? If so, I welcome you to join me on this journey towards conquering and taming the Burnout Beast.

CHAPTER ONE

THE SILENT ONSET OF BURNOUT

TRACING BURNOUT'S EMBER

I asked a couple of teenage kids I met recently what they knew about burnout and the responses I received were amazing. One described it as *'something that happened to people from working too much'* or when someone is *'no longer feeling like themselves'*. Another said *burnout was analogous to when a driver presses on the brake and accelerator at the same time and then the resultant effect is smoke!* I feel both answers are correct, with the latter describing the grave consequences that could occur when burnout is left unattended for a long time. By the time one sees smoke, there is a fire burning already.

As you can imagine, burnout doesn't just happen overnight, the telltale signs are there early on. More likely, people put a pause on some things while plowing through other tasks as though nothing were wrong, tantamount to going through the motions – almost numb, zombie-like or robo-cop-like. This leads to emotionally disconnecting from the work.

DRAINED: THE VEHICLE-BATTERY ANALOGY

Let's go back to the analogy of a driver pressing both the accelerator and brakes of a car in static motion at the same time. The car in this instance is the human body. The accelerator represents the tasks that one feels the need to fulfill even when they aren't feasible nor is it reasonable to tackle all of them at once. The brakes are the few coping tips that individuals might employ to help fix the issue. The issue is that the car – the human body – is unable to function or move in this situation. It remains static, until something gives. The early sign that all isn't well is the initial smoke, which we will call stress, and the consequence of not attending to stress soon enough is burnout. The burnout vehicle-battery analogy is further explained in Figure 1.

Let's think of stress like any battery, and assume it starts out being fully charged suggesting that one's *surge capacity* is at its maximum. Some have defined *surge capacity* as the physical and mental adaptive systems that individuals draw upon for short term survival of stressful situations[9]. The battery never runs out without warning signs; hence, surge capacity works short-term before a renewal or recharge becomes imperative. Those warning signs can be categorized into physical, emotional, and behavioral which will be addressed shortly.

STRESS AND BURNOUT

It was Eckart Tolle who described stress as *'being here but wanting to be there.'* The quote highlights both anxious and depressive symptoms associated with the impact of stress. Being in the present can be compromised by stressors. We escape stress by looking to the past or future. It is the experience that people often have when exposed to stressors (be it mild,

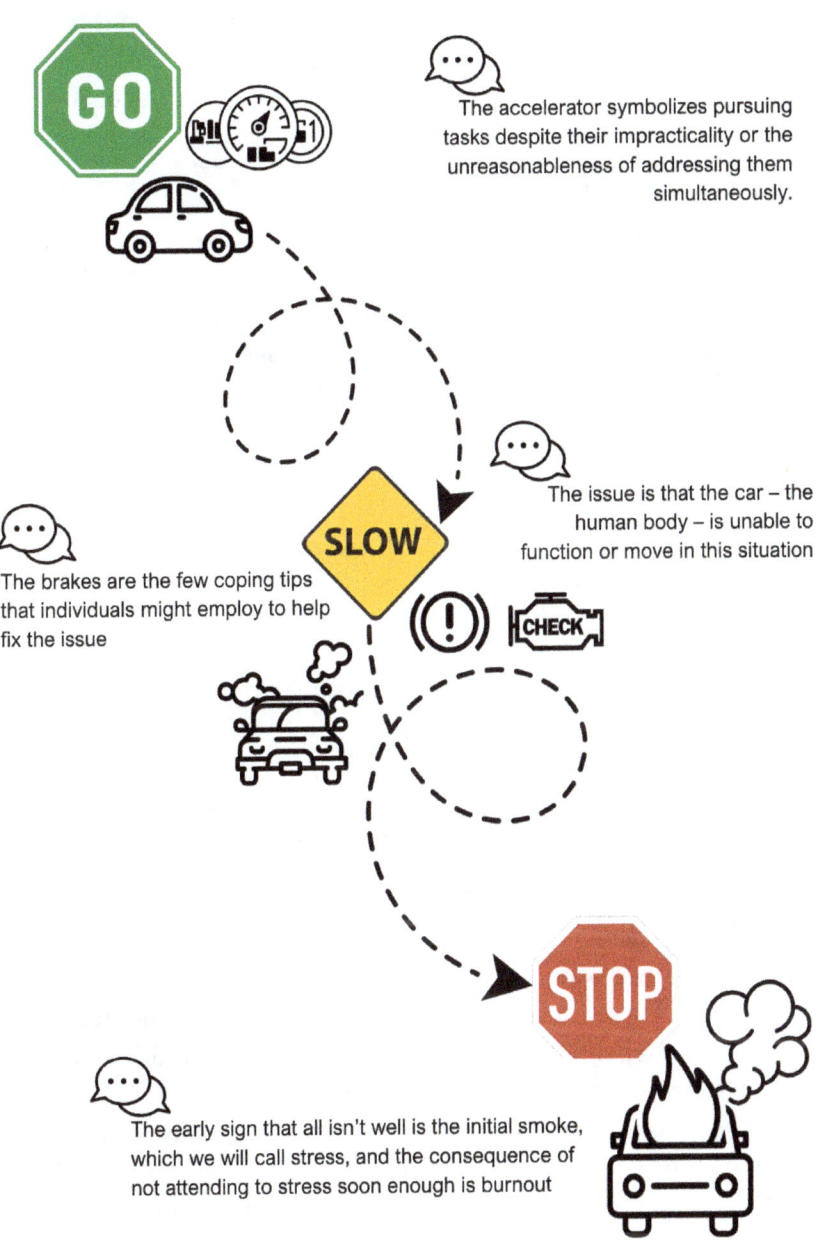

Figure 1: Burnout-Vehicle-Battery Analogy

moderate, or severe) that leads to a feeling of being put under pressure. Incidentally, it may take a while for the consequences of a mild stressor to manifest compared to a moderate or severe stressor. Mild stressors are often initially tolerable but becomes increasingly distressful over time.

It is often said that there are two types of stress, the good and the bad. Good stress is one that could be likened to challenges that are welcoming such as the number of midnight candles burned in order to gain skills or be better placed in one's current or desired career path. The sleepless nights have an expiry date to them, and so with that in mind often a tolerable inconvenience. It could be that good stress is manageable when there is a project with a high priority timeline. Team members know that the workload will sooner or later reduce as the completion milestone is achieved.

Although the purpose of this topic is about work-related stress, I will add another example of good stress. Parents of newborn often experience sleepless nights or disrupted nights but these have some end date in sight. As the newborn grows and settles into a new routine or more consistent schedule, parents are allowed some respite and more sleep. In addition to limited time, positive stress also generates joy endorphins.

Bad or negative stress on the other hand is one that has become overwhelming, with the potential to drive people to look for an outlet. These outlets are means of coping with the negative stress, and depending on which outlets accessed could either be deleterious or helpful. For example, an individual using alcohol or other psychedelic drugs to cope with work pressure is expected to have more negative consequences at work and home, while one who exercises to clear mental fog or to renew their depleted battery (energy) is doing something that has a higher chance of yielding long term positive outcomes.

Kim in 2023 explained stress and its relationship to work output, such that too much stimulation yields negative results[10].

The theory has been used by many to explain the different states of work stress, from a state of calmness to mild stress to moderate and severe stress[11]. Too little stimulation can lead to hypo-arousal in which people end up feeling bored and too much stimulation can lead to breakdown of both body and mind leading to exhaustion, burnout and so on.

Lepnurm, Dobson, Backman, and Keegan summarized these experiences into **strain**, which occurs at a lower stress spectrum, **stress** if moderate, and **burnout** if severe.[12] Our focus is on the **burnout beast**. Burnout brings with it the feeling of being overwhelmed. Bréne Brown, a seasoned social worker, describes this state of feeling overwhelmed as *'an extreme level of stress, an emotional and or cognitive intensity to the point of feeling unable to function.'*[13] That said, the inability to manage stress successfully does not rely on the individual; the society or systems, organizations, leaders and co-workers have a role to play.

MEASURING BURNOUT [6,14,15,16]

Since burnout is not a mental health condition, it is not usually measured in clinical practice. The main tool used in assessing burnout in research studies is the Maslach Burnout Inventory (MBI)[14]. There are a few versions of it, the main one being the 22- item which is more comprehensive, and a shorter version 2 item MBI that assesses emotional exhaustion (EE) that is, *"I feel burned out from my work"* and depersonalization that is *"I have become more callous toward people since I took this job"*[15]. The responses are scored on a seven-point Likert scale (0–6) with frequency of at least once a week or more often. Burnout is predictive with a score >3 for either of the two components. There are other tools like the Copenhagen Burnout Inventory or Oldenburg Burnout Inventory[15], many of which are available at a cost.

Bréne Brown says *vulnerability is not weakness; it is our greatest measure of courage*[13], and I personally couldn't agree more. Full disclosure - I have experienced burnout a few times over the last decade, with each episode different from the previous. One of the experiences occurred during my Family Medicine residency training and the other two times as an independently practicing Family Physician in Canada, with barely a four-year interval between the last two episodes. It is safe to say that burnout is something that can occur more than once in one's career, if not checked. I have also balanced empirical knowledge with my personal experiences so that you can perhaps feel connected to me as you learn to prevent or manage burnout. I believe willingness to be vulnerable and share personal experiences, even the uncomfortable ones, is crucial to guide others on the path of increasing awareness, prevention and management of burnout.

MEET AND GREET WITH BURNOUT

In 2009, Krasner and Epstein identified the occurrence of burnout among half of third year medical students and 45% of resident physicians.[16] A year after that finding was published, it dawned on me that I might be experiencing what I later found out was burnout. I was in the early stages of my residency training in Family Medicine in Canada. I honestly don't recall what came first, the chicken or the egg. My family doctor had diagnosed me with adjustment reaction and advised me to take six weeks stress leave. I was also placed on antidepressant.

Unfortunately, I was experiencing marital distress around the same time. While training, I was also raising three small children all under the age of seven. In fact, my youngest was eighteen months old when I first embarked on my journey into becoming absorbed into the field of medicine. Foreign trained medical graduates were required to go through a four-month period of training called externship. Those were unpaid periods of training. A majority of immigrant medical graduates were already struggling to keep their heads above water, and to let go of any paying menial jobs like delivering pizzas, working at gas stations or working as health care aides was adding salt to injury.

I had been privileged in my time to have some support from the health system for the period of training as a clinical assistant. That was a lifesaver, for my spouse at the time who had two engineering degrees prior to immigrating was also trying to get absorbed into the Engineering field. To say this was a rather stressful period is simply an understatement. Keep in mind that the *2021 National Physician Survey* showed that being a parent and a caregiver increased the likelihood of experiencing burnout, and being an ethnic minority, and female gender increased the likelihood that I would experience discrimination, microaggression, and intimidation.[7] Other than the caregiving role to my kids, I was also responsible for ensuring good care was being provided for my mom who had been diagnosed with a stroke and was fully dependent on others.

Let me go back a bit. My childhood dream was to live in Canada. It was quite a random dream at the time – it had nothing to do with working as a physician, or of making more money, or living larger than I would otherwise have, compared with living in Nigeria. It was simply a place my young mind desired to live in when adulthood came, which was an aspiration I had shared with my siblings as we sat around the living room in banter. At the time, I didn't know anyone who lived there. My siblings said they preferred places like America and the United Kingdom. Honestly, we did not have any reasonable yardstick with which we drew our conclusion. Simply put, we were a bunch of day-dreaming kids!

When the time finally came to relocate, I had no idea how challenging the journey would be. Prior to accepting an elective rotation in Cardiothoracic Surgery at the University of Toronto's (U of T) Sunnybrook and Women's Hospital, I met some Canadians who had offered to host me over the 1999 Christmas holidays. I had the most amazing impression of Canada during this one-month visit as a Cardiothoracic Surgery elective student. The Sunnybrook Health Sciences Centre was massive and included state-of-the-art equipment. I watched in awe as the heart-lung machine took over the function of the patient's own heart and lungs as their diseased aortic valve was being replaced with an artificial pig's during surgery. Following the procedure, I was given the opportunity to suture the incision sites with another U of T student, Trish, who was also rotating through this department. This was a very positive experience as I felt included in all the tasks each day and learned quite a lot. Was there any downside to this elective rotation? None, except that I was cured of my love for cardiothoracic surgery having experienced first-hand what the future held (early ward rounds and long operating room hours) if I were to follow that career path.

During that visit, whenever I was out in the evening with my hosts, because it was winter, the streets were lined with snow and the curbsides rather charming. To me it seemed particularly magical at night with all the Christmas decorations lighting up the streets and decking the halls and the roofs. It was an experience I relived until my return to Canada one week to Christmas in 2001. But visiting a place and residing at a place are two very different situations. With the former, the state of having no care in the world, just peace and much love was entirely possible.

Reminiscing about the wonderful Christmas I'd experienced with my hosts, I awoke to reality as 2002 rolled in. The holiday was over and if I was to survive in the land, then the daydreaming needed to stop. It was time to find my way back to medicine, the career my parents had forced me into. Well, no, it was not really *'forced'* in the true sense of the word. As early as age three, I told my parents of my interest in becoming a doctor. It was in grade eleven that I changed my mind, despite having excellent grades in my courses; which were science-focused. My dad disagreed, asking why I wanted to change my *'God-chosen career and destiny.'* It made no sense to me then, as all I cared about was that medicine wasn't my prime choice anymore. The course I was considering was pharmacy, which I felt was an equally good program.

However, everything seemed to work against my efforts to switch to Pharmacy. Maybe it was providence, but after trying multiple times without success, I resigned myself to going into medicine, thinking that the career switch needed to happen later. This made Canada more alluring.

The alternative option was to not work as hard in medical school since I would be switching courses. It was not until I failed my course examination that it dawned on me what failure felt like; a first and last for me. I had always been among the top three students in class throughout elementary and high school, so this felt quite foreign. It brought shame and guilt— it did not feel good at all. However, after grieving for a few weeks, and realizing there was still another chance to change that narrative, I resolved to get back on track. I wanted my career switch to be by choice, not because I was asked by the school to drop out of the program. So, I buckled my shoes and got back to studying, although half-heartedly. That was the first and last time I would ever fail any course. In fact, it drove me to perfectionism; nothing was good enough unless it had the stamp of honors or merit attached to it.

Medical school was stressful. Many of us drank coffee to stay awake in preparation for exams and literally burned the midnight oil each night. Many slept in study rooms rather than their beds. There was this sense of general anxiety and stress from the general perception our lecturers had at the time; the philosophy of 'you have failed until you prove otherwise'. Your guess is as good as mine as far as the medical culture and its ability to drive burnout in medical students. Sleep deprivation is a culture medical students develop early on in their training because there is just so much educational material to learn and cram for exams. Many were selected into medical schools for their high performances in high school and so the culture continues into later stages of one's medical career; manifesting as accolades and degrees (presumably the more the better).

I eventually got matched into Family Medicine Residency training and was elated, except that being unprepared for the consistent need to defend my medical education before some patients and a few preceptors, added another layer of stress on top of an already stressful training. It felt as though one needed to prove themselves repeatedly, despite having scaled all the required medical licensing examinations successfully. In fact, foreign trained medical graduates were told that based on past data, they needed to work harder if they wished to pass the Family Medicine certification examination at first try!

It appeared that the experiences of foreign-trained medical graduates (FMGs) varied from preceptor to preceptor. Although recency of practice also varied among the FMGs, some have more training and experience than the average medical graduate would have had going into residency. The closest I came to having someone question my competency was during my Internal Medicine rotation at a very busy hospital in the city. The issue was that after being on call for twenty-four hours straight, I was still expected to perform at my best the next morning at rounds with the preceptor assigned for the week. Much as I had struggled to stay awake to review the patient's condition and differential diagnoses, my brain was on autopilot. My brain refused to do as I bid it; it was just not cooperating with me, in terms of retaining the required information for rounds purposes.

Not surprisingly, I didn't provide the correct answer to a question on electrolyte imbalance caused by Syndrome of Inappropriate Antidiuretic Hormone (SIADH) and that was the end! One strike and you are out. No chance to redeem myself following that interaction; in fact, it seemed I was no longer part of the rounds for the rest of the morning before heading home. This unfortunate event was the last impression the preceptor had of me since his week ended that day. With the new preceptor, I was on call over the weekend and ran the show. My evaluation at the end of the rotation was very positive, which was a relief.

To put this mildly, some foreign trained medical graduates report being treated unfairly by some people in the health system. Before the start of rotations, it is easy to predict which rotations are likely to be problematic based on peers' experiences. That's not to say that those assumptions were accurate, but they were certainly anxiety-provoking. Many become, *"Yes, Sir"* or *"Yes, Ma'am"* type of people; people-pleasers, to avoid problems.

Anyway, the point here is that behaviors like bullying, harassment, and micro-aggressions are burnout triggers[7], particularly when the exposure is prolonged. Recall that the home front was not doing well either, so this was a very fitting combination for what seemed like a perfect storm! The difficulty in the marriage was the straw that broke the camel's back, as is often the case. A person might be better able to handle toxic work situations if the home front is rock solid in terms of support.

After what seemed like ages, I mustered the courage to see my family doctor. I had registered to be part of this individual's patient panel prior to being offered a spot for residency training. Following that visit, and despite my hesitation, he graciously gave me a sick note to present to the program director. The truth; I was overwhelmed. I was exhausted. It was very difficult for me to get out of bed in the morning. Nonetheless, I still had to go through the motions for my family, and not so much myself. The plan of becoming an independently practicing family physician in the community meant there was no time for slowing down or stopping part way through my training.

The other challenge I had was *sickness-presenteeism,*[17] which meant that even though I was not at my best, I had to show up to care for my assigned patients. The thought of taking six weeks off of my training was something I couldn't imagine doing, *even though I needed it.* And this was despite having disrupted sleep and feeling unrefreshed each morning.

After taking some time off my training, I was able to spend some time in deep reflection of what laid ahead. And although the situation at home had not eased either, I was able to focus and was energized again after making the decision that my happiness was not for others to determine. Choosing to listen to my inner self; the thought that I was enough became a mantra of sorts. Additionally, I felt armed for independent practice at the end of my training, particularly as my research project was on Burnout Review in Family Physicians. I knew the dos and don'ts, so to speak.

The point being that personal factors like compulsive personality traits and neuroticism predispose people to burnout, that 'an inherent drive to keep going with failure to recognize one's limits[16]. This eventually leads to the phenomenon *'sickness-presenteeism'*, whereby minor health problems are ignored despite the awareness that taking sick leave is necessary. Unfortunately, this phenomenon is not entirely an intrinsic or personal issue, considering colleagues and the society place high expectations on physicians, thereby encouraging a false sense of invisibility.[17]

This is another breeding ground for shame and blame from being seen as 'not tough enough' or 'too weak' or 'not resilient' giving rise to the beginnings of isolating ourselves from reaching out for help. The other stressors that increase the risk of burnout include type of specialty (e.g. Family Medicine, Emergency Medicine and Internal Medicine), and being a caregiver to children under age twenty-one.[15,1]

I overworked and barely had any time for self.

Alas! Despite all I knew about burnout and prolonged stress, it appears the rules around how high my plate was allowed to pile up had been forgotten. By 2019, I recall experiencing some level of burnout. This time, I had all the signs in the three main domains: *physical, emotional, and behavioral.*

I already had sleep challenges from being on call 24 hours every day for ten years while working with seniors. This was the case despite there being an existing on-call after hours system in place. From continuity of care and inappropriate hospital transfer perspectives, like some others, being there for my patients round-the-clock reduces challenges for the physician on-call who doesn't know the patients. The team members loved the easy access, despite being irritable from being called too many times overnight for non-urgent matters.

For this reason, my phone was always by my bedside from the year 2011 until 2021. Imagine being sleep deprived for a decade! Some have linked sleep deprivation with consequences like medical errors, increased irritability, anxiety, fatigue, and burnout. I experienced these at different points.

So, for someone who was already experiencing sleep challenges, receiving a letter from the college regarding a patient complaint was not part of the plan at all. I became anxious about the future of my practice, all the while continuing to practice as though all was well. I confided in a few people – friends and family. I had trouble understanding what had gone wrong. It was hard not to think about the medical error on a day-to-day basis. Every email from the college thereafter made me panic, and the longer it took for the college to complete its review process, the worse my anxiety grew, out of fear of a potential doomsday.

Honestly, I didn't think this was a case of over-reacting. I felt my means of livelihood was at stake, on top of all the hoops and loops I had to go through to get into the medical field in Canada. In retrospect, I admit to being overworked with barely any time for self-care. The complaint was legitimate in some respects. I did not write a detailed note of what had transpired at the said visit. In fact, from the little I had written, I wondered if I had taken the pain to listen to the patient. I went to my usual detail-oriented self again, not allowing myself to get distracted.

In retrospect, I admit to being overworked with barely any time for self-care. While fully immersed in my full-time practice, I simultaneously embarked on two distinct graduate-level programs, all while fulfilling the responsibilities of a caregiver at home! So what really happened that forced me to stop working the way I was? It wasn't the college complaint. This speaks to the invincibility factor we hear about.

We talked about good stress being something desirable earlier in this chapter. The problem is that good stress, when prolonged, is a good recipe for burnout as well. The desire for another challenge than what I was used to in practice, led to enrolling in two post-graduate programs. While it is always a great idea to improve one's knowledge and skills, tackling it at the same time as full time work was to my detriment. I could have taken those courses one at a time, with enough intervals between.

Most doctors and others in the health field often forget that they are not super-human. When the brake pad is already worn and due for a change, one continues to drive the car as though it could never succumb or have brake failure on the highway. Unfortunately, the pandemic also caused healthcare providers to continue to show up at work because hospitals were at capacity, and they could not have the needed time off work for several weeks to months as they were used to. Not good.

What made me finally slow down? It was the physical symptoms of burnout that had developed from wear and tear related to repetitive hand, elbow, and shoulder movements while using the computer in writing notes. On this fateful day, I had showed up at the clinic and was going through the motions by providing care to my patients when it finally hit me: the pain in my elbow, shoulder, and wrist was totally unbearable. The pain killers I had taken moments before did nothing for the pain. It had reached a height.

This realization made me decide on the spot that indeed I had had enough and did not have anything left to give that day. Unfortunately for my patients, I had to cancel the rest of the clinic day. Those who had seen me earlier that day felt sorrier for me than they did for themselves, as I grappled with guilt feelings around the inconvenience of not fulfilling my obligation to them as their family doctor. I really had no other options because the affected areas were swollen and very sore.

My physical body was collapsing, even though I was still emotionally managing to keep Body and Soul together. This time around it was easier to piece all the signs and symptoms of burnout together, confirming I was again experiencing burnout. There's also the unspoken expectation to see a minimum volume of patients per clinic day, due to the clinic expenses that physicians need to contribute towards from month to month. This is not making excuses, although it might appear that way.

Recall that stress when unchecked can cause physical, emotional and behavioral symptoms. Gabor Mate, in his book *'When the Body Says No: the Hidden Cost of Stress'*[18] eloquently described the chronic pain and other autoimmune diseases that have been linked to chronic stress and its resultant chronic inflammation. The inflammation arises from hormones and chemicals like cortisol and adrenaline that the brain releases in the context of stress and burnout which manifest physically.

The physical burnout symptoms linked with the release of adrenaline include faster heart rates and high blood pressure, and cortisol release associated with diabetes and chronic pain, with chronic exhaustion another example of physical symptom. Some of the psychological and emotional signs of burnout include mental fogginess, or decreased self-esteem, guilt, cynicism, pessimism, frustration, mistrust, mood swings, or mood changes like anxiety or depression.

Some behavioral changes that manifest are chronic complaining, absenteeism, drug addiction, overprescribing medications due to preference for avoiding any confrontation with patients, medical and nursing errors, indifference, excessive criticism of self and others.[10] There are other unintended consequences such as a decrease in patient safety and quality of care being provided, college complaints related to medical errors, and early retirement or reduced workload[11]. *'Living in disequilibrium or living dysregulated and loss of contentment equals loss of gratitude or the state of calm where we live optimally'*, as my friend Susan Hastie, a psychologist put it.

Eventually I made the hard decision to let go.

Having considered all my options, including the fact that I could not use my right hand or elbow for activities like driving or typing for prolonged hours, stepping away from clinical work for a few months was the only sane thing to do. After a while, I retuned to part-time work to avoid worsening or recurrence of combination of bursitis and tendinitis in addition to hand weakness from ulnar nerve damage from unknown cause.

That year, I felt that there *was 'nothing left to give'*. I was constantly emotionally exhausted, my physical energy level severely depleted and also from a system that no longer felt very welcoming no matter how hard I worked. I was beginning to doubt myself and my abilities because of a few local work-culture issues that led to excessive workload, lack of control or input in matters relating to patient care, inefficient work processes, and clerical burdens[11]. It felt as though I was 'not enough' which of course isn't true at all.

It was at an Instagram live session with a colleague that I was reminded of the impact of COVID-19 pandemic with political decisions made around remuneration that negatively impacted the morale of a lot of physicians. She listed what she felt was the outcome of those decisions—some family physicians left for other provinces, some early retirement and yet others modified their practices in significant ways. In that same year, many medicine residency training offers remained unfilled country-wide.

She shared that medical students are not enthusiastic about going into the field of Family Medicine. Family medicine used to be a specialty where physicians feel a connection with their patients from birth to elderly stages of life, including end of life in many instances. Family physicians are front liners and gatekeepers, by virtue of their roles which include treating diverse ailments, time pressure to keep clinic flow, large amounts of paperwork, delays in getting specialist inputs and general sense of feeling undervalued oft cited for contributing to stress and burnout. [4,17]

For many, this work counts as fulfilling one's calling, but sooner or later there will likely be negative interactions from peers or patients that leave many pondering whether the field is as fulfilling as it once was. Physicians are high functioning individuals who don't take kindly to medical errors[12], despite the realization that they are human. Consequences of burnout or medical errors include anxiety or depression, substance use and a few have lost their lives to suicide.[11] What one might never find out is whether burnout was the precursor to dying by suicide, or other factors..

Personally, despite exercising more, eating healthy meals and practicing mindfulness as part of my de-stressing strategies, the feeling of exhaustion did not budge much. The more self-reflection I did, the more the realization that my workload needed further modification for me to feel better on a longer term. I realized yet again that something needed to give. Eventually I made the hard decision to let go of my clinical work, despite modifying my work load every so often.

I must admit though that each time I reduced my clinical duties; the proportion of my non-clinical work increased. So, I did not tackle the workload issue properly. The other drivers of burnout in my case were working with a patient population with very high complex needs, commuting to a smaller town two hours per commute for two years.

My story need not be yours since highlighting some of the burnout drivers are aimed at helping you recognize and manage it better.

REFLECTION QUESTIONS
LET'S MAKE A PLAN

It is much easier to prevent burnout than manage its consequences.

1. Using the two item Maslach Burnout Inventory: Are you experiencing emotional exhaustion or signs of depersonalization, if so how often?
2. Have you experienced burnout in the last month? In what domains of burnout do you currently identify with? How about in the past?
3. Can you please write down what they look like now and or in the past?
4. Do you know of anyone, colleague or friend or family member who might have symptoms that appear like burnout?
5. What would it take to approach someone you think might be burned out; to genuinely ask if they are doing okay?
6. What plans have you made for rainy day? Example, if you were forced to take time off work due to burnout; to reset?
7. Do you have disability insurance; long or short term in the event your health takes a tumble? Is the type of insurance you currently have it adequate to meet inflation needs and those of your immediate family, if any?

CHAPTER TWO

THE CULPRIT WITHIN

CULTURE CREATES BURNOUT

This chapter aims to discuss burnout drivers using the lens of culture.

Merriam Webster dictionary defines culture *as 'the customary beliefs, social forms, and material traits of a racial, religious, or social group.'*[19] It also goes on to explain it as *'the set of shared attitudes, values, goals, and practices that characterizes an institution or organization'.*

When carefully assessed, it seems to me that culture has the potential to drive perfection which can inevitably increase burnout risks. No human being can perform at their best every single day, neither can machines perform at their best every day, without ongoing maintenance. According to Susan Hastie, *'perfectionism is in fact an unachievable standard, which is why the bar keeps getting raised every so often'.* Often, the systems we find ourselves in dictate the pace and work expectations, which in turn impacts us at all levels, professionally and personally. Systems (for example governments, and regulatory bodies) set expectations which are geared towards the public good. However, these expectations are expressed through policies that influence organizational positions and stances which ultimately affect workers. It is noteworthy to mention that systemic changes are often the result of high expectations from the public as well. These expectations create a demand and pressure for performance from top to bottom[17]. These expectations influence what we know and call industry or workplace culture.

While there is nothing inherently wrong with having policies, rules, and regulations for industries, organizations, and workers, when these are not in balance with checks and processes that evaluate outcomes, it is easy to become blind-sighted. It need not remain this way. An organization or system that embraces a culture of a holistic approach to its programs and services will excel and outlast competitors. The markers for success are high-quality products, programs, and services, client and worker satisfaction, to name a few.

Perhaps let's start with identifying some of the cultural barriers (also summarized in Figure 2) as a way of informing the needed change. Culture will be subdivided into three layers: system (industry), organizational (workplace), and personal.

SYSTEM CULTURE AS A BURNOUT DRIVER

Note that as you read, I will make an attempt to categorize systems versus industry culture as separate entities, there will remain some overlap.

The idea of system or organizational culture as burnout drivers cannot be overemphasized, hence the focus on this early on in this book. If there is one message I would encourage you to take away from reading this chapter, it is to know that burnout is often work-related. It is the culture from the top to bottom that has the biggest impact on a person's wellbeing than individual factors.

Also, important to note at the outset that individual or personal factors can contribute to a higher burnout risk, particularly if the organization itself has not effectively addressed issues bordering on workers' wellness. For example, top-down approaches[20] to policy changes or lack of transparency, inequitable remuneration, inadequate staffing, lack of wellness programs or a culture that encourages wellness, leaders who do not adopt *trauma-informed* approaches in their interactions with workers, lack of sense of belonging from workplaces that may well be diverse but remain non-inclusive, or lack of worker appreciation to name a few. See the definition of *trauma* and *trauma-informed* in the glossary.

Organizations that strictly focus on client or patient satisfaction, without commensurate emphasis on the wellness and wellbeing of worker have imbibed cultures that are harmful. This stance is tantamount to an worker having value only when leaders, clients or patients rate workers' performance as good. Many workers might coast along for a while without frequent positive feedback from the systems they find themselves in; but I surmise that it is only a question of time before strain sets in, followed by moderate stress which when becomes severe leads to burnout. Workers are more likely to describe their work environments as toxic if their sense of self-worth is questioned or interactions with others are often negative, or opportunities for wellness are lacking in the workplace. It appears that some organizations are satisfied provided workers do not complain about system deficiencies, continue to show up to work with a false sense of wellbeing, even if they were slowly buckling down physically and mentally. This would be a culture that encourages a lack of authenticity, something I will call **Work COLA** (a culture of a lack of authenticity). It's like a ticking time bomb. The detonation of the bomb represents the point at which systems and leaders are forced to rethink the status quo.

One thing remains clear - regardless of the system, governments or organizations that do not invest in their workers wellness, will in time, pay quite dearly for periods of worker neglect, whatever the neglect might be.

ORGANIZATIONAL CULTURE: BURNOUT'S ALLY

It appears that depending on one's field of career there are high expectations; the demands organizations put on people. This high expectation starts early on, from training days all the way to more advanced career stages. From entry into the universities with high grade point average (GPA) or scores, to long duration of training, and the higher in the career path one gravitates, the higher the expectation becomes. Many attribute success to longer duration of training, higher qualifications and academic achievements with grades like merit or honors which further drive the high achiever to over-perform or outperform others.

Remuneration is often graded, with highest paid typically those with the highest qualifications, although this is not always the case. An individual might have a law degree and choose to switch careers. For some immigrants, switching careers is often not a choice matter, rather a necessity from having to deal with *'Canadian Experience'* limitations. This simply means that though they have equivalent degrees and certifications with Canadian counterparts, they are unable to land jobs in the Canadian work environment due to lack of Canadian experience. Many resort to volunteering to gain experience and taking menial jobs to keep head above water. In most cases, they take a pay cut and are unable to live as well as they once did, particularly for those who were engineers, doctors, nurses, or lawyers in their countries of birth.

I will give an example. After relocating to Canada, almost every job I applied for was met with what I will call **OQCE** which is *'over qualification without Canadian experience'*. I then took a job as an administrative staff that also performed blood draws and took patient histories. It paid about the minimum wage. This organization hired immigrant physicians only for this position, knowing that they would get skilled labour for cheap.

These immigrants were also less likely to complain about the pay inequity since many would not otherwise be able to put food on the table for their families. Although the pay at the time barely did much for me, given I could only work part-time due to the office set-up that was built around specialist availability and the fact that I was also attending full time classes in Clinical Research, I was glad to be somewhat self-sufficient. This is not about ingratitude to a system that opened the door to me or others. It isn't about blame either. The point being made here isn't that Canada is a horrible place to live in or that it doesn't treat immigrants fairly.

On the contrary, being the country of my childhood dreams I love it with all my heart, and there's no place I'd rather be. The goal is improvement. And yes, while my initial journey was tough and very challenging due to some of the policies in place at the time of immigration, I do not wish to live anywhere else. Yes, even during winter months. I find winter can be captivating and magical, especially around Christmas. And after twenty years in Canada, I am yet to consider becoming a snowbird; at least not yet.

PERFECTIONISM: THE TALENT TRAP

Among American ethnic minority university faculty, there were significant racial differences in burnout prevalence at a third for the early career under-represented ethnic minority groups compared to their white (18%) and Asian (3%) counterparts.[13]

Many organizations many pay attention to additional achievements and training beyond a first degree and reward their workers based on higher educational levels. This causes some inequity issues; for instance, the worker with a learning disability or financial constraint that prevents them from investing in higher education or additional skill-enhancing certifications may be disadvantaged in the ability to better self. Disenfranchisement occurs from remaining in the system that pays no attention to long years of service without any consideration for advancement.

Despite the additional training and certification that some possess, it appears their race, gender, sexual orientation, religious beliefs, or disability has placed them in a disadvantageous position. I have heard many such anecdotes shared amongst ethnic minority groups[1] in which their colleagues rise through the ranks more easily, whereas they need to prove why they merit a leadership position. Few are encouraged to apply for leadership positions, and when they do, barely make it to perfunctory interview round than true quest for both diversity and inclusion. Sometimes the hiring processes within organizations are flawed, and that talents are lost based on conscious and unconscious biases. It behooves everyone to be more mindful of these potential barriers and finds ways to mitigate them. Implicit or explicit biases have been known to drive physician burnout.

For those in the medical field, the Hippocratic Oaths medical students swear upon graduation which idealizes the role of the physician could also be one of the major drivers fueling the sense of invincibility that physicians adopt. Like cultists, physicians swear to that oath, which not only attests to *'do no harm'*, but also puts all else before self, the difference being this is publicly declared and it impacted my life from that day on. There is nothing wrong with people pledging to uphold the profession or being accountable for care they provide to society members; in fact it is laudable.

The overarching goal of the oath being to *'do no harm'*, except that the high burnout rates in physicians could be linked with the heightened sense of invincibility that the oath they swore to create. This is one aspect of societal expectation of who a doctor should be. The badge of honor comes with spending over 60 hours a week on the job, as do lawyers, or accountants during tax season especially. *Sometimes what is needed is a keen candidate or worker with a mixture of strong educational background and experiences, with a little more support from the organization to achieve their maximum potential, thereby reducing job mismatch issues.*

Whether unionized or not, remuneration issues have the potential to impact people's well-being negatively. Policies can have unintended effects that contribute to a sense of lack of appreciation in workers which can negatively impact the sense of professional fulfillment that people have towards the work they do.

Other factors like inflation and economic downturns do not help the situation. This reality drives the inability of people to effectively cope with their basic needs of life such that some work two or more jobs to make ends meet. Sometimes working two or more jobs helps individuals meet not just their own needs but those of extended or nuclear family locally or abroad. This is especially true for immigrant families, thereby increasing the risk of burnout in these individuals.

SYSTEM DRIVERS

CULTURAL
- High expectation from industry driving culture of invincibility and sickness presenteeism
- Too much client focus & non-prioritization of employee wellness
- Culture of saying little (ineffective communication)
- A lack of worker appreciation, disrespectful and harmful approaches during restructuring

LACK OF INNOVATION & CREATIVITY
- Utilizing non-objective measurements
- Tunnel vision
- Top-down approaches
- Ineffective forecasting mechanism

POLITICS & POLICIES
- Non-inclusive and Inequitable policies
- Accountability issues
- Non-transparency
- Human Resource Unit privy to leader-worker issues creating bias
- Mistrust issues
- Ostrich stance

REMUNERATION ISSUES
- Utilizing outdated pay-grade scales in the face of inflation
- Culture of undervaluation of worker skills and trainings

ORGANIZATIONAL

CULTURAL
- Non-inclusive cultures: 'us vs. them'; Work COLA, lack of promotion of worker self-agency

WORKER SUPPORT ISSUES
- Inequitable approaches used in supporting the marginalized, under-represented (e.g people with disability)

MISMATCH ISSUES
- Non-alignment of leadership roles and decision-making authority
- Work-employee job mismatch

WORK ENVIRONMENT ISSUES (TOXIC WORKPLACES)
- Lack of worker appreciation
- Violence and assaults: sexual and non-sexual (physical)
- Policies and procedures that allow conscious and unconscious bias thrive: racism and discrimination
- Gossiping
- Micro-aggressions, bullying and harassment

LEADERSHIP ISSUES
- Communication issues: too little or ineffective communication driving mistrust, cynicism, disengagement
- Micro-management
- Ill-equipped leaders
- Autocratic leadership styles
- Faulty worker Periodic Review processes

PERSONAL

FAMILY CULTURE
- Individualist vs. collectivist
- Unrealistic expectations of family members regarding assuming career roles, career choices (future expectations

CHILDHOOD EXPERIENCES
- Trauma (abuse, neglect)
- Intimate partner violence
- Sense of worth
- Resilience

RELATIONSHIP DIFFICULTIES
- Divorce
- Parent-teen, or parent-adult child challenges
- Separation
- Death

PERSONALITY & BEHAVIOUR ISSUES
- Difficulty setting boundaries
- Perfectionism
- People Pleasing
- Work-life imbalance (workaholism)

HARMFUL LIFESTYLES
- Substance abuse: narcotic prescriptions, recreational drugs (cocaine, amphetamines), marijuana, alcohol
- Unhealthy relationship with food and beverages

Figure 2: A Comprehensive Review of Culture & Burnout Drivers

ORGANIZATIONAL CULTURE: BURNOUT'S PLAYGROUND

In my opinion, the nursing profession does a better job at creating a healthier culture than medicine does, with such simple steps like protected break times, belonging to unions, encouraging internal social events. That said, when there is a crisis, the last thing a nurse would be thinking of is to take a well deserved break. Nurses are less likely to have a real break on a consistent basis, since to expect calmness during their shifts each day is outright unrealistic. They have multiple tasks they must perform from shift to shift. From training others, providing medications or care to patients, to performing procedures like inserting or changing out urinary or gastrointestinal catheters or for those in tertiary hospital systems more sophisticated monitoring of the vital signs of patients such as oxygen levels, heart rates and breathing rates required to keep patients in critical conditions alive. Since the pandemic, studies after studies highlight the rather high burnout rates at over one in two, especially young female nurses.[14]

The COVID-19 viral outbreak brought with it a need for full donning- and-doffing personal protective wears or equipment to prevent healthcare workers from contracting the virus. They are the ones who have more consistent and closest contact with patients or clients, depending on their work settings. Since this book is being written just post-pandemic, reference to the situation is unavoidable, as this was a time when most healthcare workers and other essential service workers were stretched thin and beyond their usual capacity.

As a nursing home primary care provider and medical director of a care home, I volunteered to be one of the designated Covid- physicians for the site, meaning I and another colleague provided in-person care to residents who had been diagnosed with the virus, while the other physicians provided virtual care to decrease contact and spread of the virus.

With how fast-spreading and rapidly-mutating the virus was, it is no surprise therefore that the resultant high burnout rate remains an ongoing issue, even outside healthcare. The pandemic brought more challenges like reduced workforce from viral illness and other physical or mental health issues that may or may not be directly linked with prolonged stress or burnout. Let's explore the experience of Carla, from Poland, a nurse with over twenty years' experience.

CARLA THE NURSE

I will highlight some of the organizational issues that led to burnout for Carla based on her account and my understanding of what transpired. Carla recalled several work situations in which she was beginning to *feel disenfranchised* whenever she showed up at work. The same feeling was absent outside of work settings. She was nostalgic about the good old days when there was light snacks in the staff lunchroom, enough workers for assigned work and a clean and more welcoming work environment. What had changed *was inadequate staffing* with less staff performing work that needed more hands without commensurate increase in remuneration, the discontinuation and restriction of much needed resources required for optimal performance of daily tasks attributed to cost concerns on the part of the organization.

Regarding her organization's expectations for her *roles and responsibilities*, she felt there was a *mismatch*. She was being tasked with training newly hired staff members as the longest serving staff in the organization even though that was not in her job description. That aside, she noticed that when her colleagues called in sick, there was an *unspoken mandate for her to hold the fort* until either an agency staff was recruited or another staff member volunteer to cover that shift. Her *work hours had also been changed several times without much notice* to her.

It was harder for her to get away for medical appointments and attend to health needs, whereas this was a non-issue in the past with her previous leaders. She began to book medical appointments as late in the day as possible that the doctor's office could permit. Also, due to the newly mandated work hours she had not agreed to, she found she was exhausted most evenings and no longer able to go for walks after dinner or even enjoy hiking like she once did. The energy was simply not there, no matter how much rest she got on her days off!

Carla shared that she no longer felt a sense of belonging within her organization, as the workplace also saw a **very high turnover rate across board.** And belonging is innate to everyone's survival. The new senior leader had scrapped off some of the perks the staff received in the past which contributed to the pride in belonging to the organization. She recounted the innumerable times the facility she worked out of was on one outbreak or the other, such as stomach flu. This meant that nurses spent more time donning on and doffing off their personal protective equipment (**PPE**), which led to tasks taking longer than is expected during shifts. There was also a reduction or lack of much needed lunch or coffee breaks, and a shortening of the expected routine time off because of fears around job loss if they refused longer or extra shifts.

Many times, nursing staff also share that they carry a sense of heavy guilt when they think about the needs of the residents they care for and the potential negative outcomes to their clients if they did not pick up shifts to help out. This arises from relationships that healthcare workers build with their clients or patients, and not a failure on the organization's part.

She expressed a similar sense of guilt around taking needed time off work, despite the **unsupportive worker wellness** policies. *Walking the talk is central to worker wellness.* This can be promoted by gestures as little as giving staff the permission to attend to their health and wellbeing. She gave an instance of a time when she called in sick at work and the very next day her immediate supervisor phoned her asking when she was returning to work. She did not feel that her recovery mattered or was paramount to her leader compared with the desire to fulfill a work need. Due to worry about job insecurity in the context of a downturn in the global economy which could negatively impact her retirement, Carla was back to work the next day. In addition to the listed fears, she felt guilty while off sick and worried about disappointing her colleagues who would have to work longer hours to ensure adequate coverage of the facility. The challenge with providing adequate staffing sometimes is that agencies do not always have a worker available for certain shifts, plus facilities' preferences for a regular staff worker because of the familiarity with their processes and expectations.

The Role of Colleagues

For all her hard work and conscientiousness, she felt she often received negative feedback from her supervisors. It seemed that the only time she heard from them was when things went bad. For this organization, **feedback imbalance** seems to be an issue for Carla's manager. Worker feedback processes, formal and informal, should be balanced with ongoing regular appreciation for hard work and dedication and a culture of improvement and support when there are gaps. Carla was not expecting a pay raise. Although for the work she performed each day, a raise would have been appropriate. An organizational culture lacking in worker recognition and wellness,especially in settings where witnessing death and dying, with potentially higher risks for moral distress, example, healthcare, is a burnout driver .

Sometimes the issue ***is unrealistic expectations from colleagues***. For example, when short staffed, Carla's colleagues expected her to slide in and assume a more junior role upon being made aware of a staffing situation which meant switching gears from junior leader position to frontline staff at the drop of a hat. This would totally be alright for Carla; except they occurred many times each week for months and years.

The eye-opener for Carla was during an interaction with her when I noticed she was using clauses like *'I don't care. I don't care anymore'* repeatedly. She was constantly showing up at work, but she was not present, a situation itself with potential for grave consequences. I carefully informed Carla that she might be experiencing burnout, and she was taken aback. She had wondered why she was feeling the way she had been for a long time. This knowledge helped her take a step back to address some of her challenges. I will share some of these in another chapter.

Carla's experiences of high job-related stress corresponds to those reported by authors like Stordeu who found that nurses with perceptions of high job demand and lower level of control, conflicts with co-workers or physicians, more frequent death and dying of patients were at higher risk of experiencing burnout[21].

The negative consequences to organizations is low motivation and performance that can extend to cause a reduction in the quality of services, causing greater conflicts, emotional "contagion effect", generating a toxic working environment and significant economic losses through absenteeism, loss of efficiency or counterproductive behaviors.[14]

KAI THE BUSINESS ANALYST

Burnout spares no profession, although it is commoner in some such as the health sector. Let me briefly share another burnout story from another client's perspective. This client, who I will call Kai, had something many have. **People-pleasing**. People-pleasing that is excessive can lead to **emotional exhaustion** and **neglect** of their own needs. For Kai, he felt **overwhelmed and was very frustrated** from failed attempts at deciphering what was wrong with him. He described having daily chronic headaches in work settings and severe fatigue at the end of each workday that the only energy he had left was just enough to eat dinner and he would slump into bed, only to wake up the next morning, having gone to bed around 7 pm. He felt he had nothing left in him to give to his family members. He was beginning to have **outbursts at work** and was **more irritable.**

Burnout had changed his personality. He is not a bad person at all; he has a kind heart. He could not understand why **no one else understood** him. How come no one could see that he was nearing a nervous breakdown? How come no one understood that this was his cry for help? His plate was already full, but despite that it seemed his **organization's priorities were constantly changing.** He felt torn between his passion for his work and the excessive demand placed on him by his boss and colleagues as they wanted him to drop the work he was tackling to immediately attend to their needs, often ***without much notice or room for a dialogue on reasonable turnaround time.*** The worst part was that those he felt could do something to help him were compounding things for him at work. This left him ***feeling trapped***, despite an appreciation for the perks workers got as benefits working for the said organization.

Burnout the beast was doing a number on him. And it seemed it did not take much for him to be triggered, as a negative way of coping to try and protect what was left of him. Remember he had nothing more to give at this stage? Stress expressed through cynicism (emotional), mistakes (behavioral), creates an easily triggered worker who, when activated protects himself from burning out further. Hence, what was once used for connecting with others, belonging as it were, is now used to conserve; protect self against burnout. The negative result is that the curiosity and interest in learning on the job diminishes as protecting against further workplace stress becomes the focus.

Kai appeared to be more frustrated because he had been attending counselling with a paid therapist when he met me. Kai began therapy when he first noticed he was experiencing **mental fogginess.** He was at a point where he felt that **'people think I'm crazy'**, and to crown it all, **'I can't recognize myself'**. His work performance was declining, although it was not apparent to others, and while others praised his work, he knew he was struggling. He came to me for counselling help after several months of feeling this way, with an agreement that after two sessions if he didn't feel he was getting the needed help he was free to move on.

First, Kai was raised in Malaysia and migrated to Canada about two decades earlier. Kai worked his way through the ranks and held a position in an oil and gas company of repute. His salary was great, money was not an issue. He was always **promised salary raises whenever it seemed to his boss that he might quit** on him. The most recent promise was that the company would pay for him to get a post graduate degree if he so desired, and a promotion but he declined that offer knowing he was struggling.

It was several months later that things got worse. He had sought help from his family doctor and then therapist. It seemed no one could tell him exactly what was wrong with him. No one was offering a solution that was targeting the exhaustion and overwhelming feeling he felt. He felt he had done all he could to get his life back on track, but nothing was working. This was despite eating healthy, exercising daily, attending physiotherapy sessions for his chronic muscular pain and using home remedies for sleep problems. According to Kai, his therapist told him that his boss was not the issue, but his work habits. Kai was at a loss for words; he became more desperate for solutions.

He was at a loss for words; he became more desperate seeking solutions. Kai shared that his frustration was that he was regularly asked to take on roles outside of his job description. Kai said he did not mind the job demands, except the turnaround time fo the delivery of work was unrealistic. His job required that he collaborated with multiple stakeholders and making new connections on the fly, which left him ***feeling disorganized and he felt a loss of control of self-agency***.

He was unable to deliver as efficiently as he once did due to the body aches and pain he had developed. At a point he also felt that God had abandoned him, although he continued to be spiritually inclined. If anyone ever noticed that he was struggling, it was not mentioned; a situation that was like an **'ostrich effect'** described by others, where leaders or organization fail to take necessary steps to address the status quo.

Kai's boss was supportive of his work at first, but he had begun to question the toxic worker-worker interactions that appeared to go unnoticed by his boss. For instance, tackling multiple unrelated tasks, non-collaborative work practices, non-trauma-informed leadership approaches, have the potential to negatively impact worker health and negatively, leading to burnout. Some organizations and leaders do not demonstrate the prioritization of worker wellbeing when unwell, despite providing workplace fitness of wellness areas.

CHAPTER THREE

THE DOMINO EFFECT

PEOPLE-PLEASING TO PERISHING

No one can understand the intricacies and outcome of any movie by fast-forwarding to the very end. This chapter aims to present some of the ways that burnout has presented itself in real people; professionals in various fields and the list aren't exhaustive. The purpose of sharing clients' burnout stories is to provide concrete examples that might stimulate you to reflect on your own feelings and experiences and identify potential similarities or differences with one or more of these individuals.

These individuals, who are like you and I in so many ways, did not experience burnout because they were 'weak' or 'not resilient enough'. They experienced burnout due to chronic pleasing, which means giving of themselves to the point of near-death. Yes, indeed, burnout could lead to death, if unattended. That bias regarding 'not being tough enough' goes as far as perpetuating stigma and silence about burnout which prevents people from seeking the help they need. The key point here is that regardless of the burnout phase one is at; example, early, mid or late phases, it isn't too late to take charge of ones health and wellness lifeboat. *Taking charge of your health and wellness lifeboat involves taking the captain's corner, steering the boat toward wellness despite the turbulence created by the winds or the waves.*

Before we delve into the personal stories and the cultural factors at play, let's start with a recap of the science regarding chronic stress and their resultant effects on the brain. Various anatomy, embryology and physiology books show the parts of the brain, their evolution and how they function.

Three main parts of the brain to keep in mind for understanding how the brain responds to stress are the prefrontal cortex, the amygdala and the hippocampus (the learning and memory centre) as seen on Figure 3. The *prefrontal cortex (PFC)* is responsible for making meaning of things (rationalization), decision-making, abstract reasoning, insight, language and also inhibits inappropriate social behavior[22]. Its functioning depends on a state of alertness, meaning that if someone is experiencing fatigue or uncontrollable stress, the PFC goes 'offline' through series of chemical events that lead to the disconnection of the brain (neural) circuits, which *'weaken'* the PFC function.[22] These chemicals are also released in the amygdala (a part of the more primitive brain responsible for fear and emotions), which causes the 'strengthening' of the unconscious habits and emotional responses.[22] This means that when people feel the stress they are handling is manageable; the PFC inhibits the stress response such that those chemicals are not released, thereby maintaining a balanced brain environment.

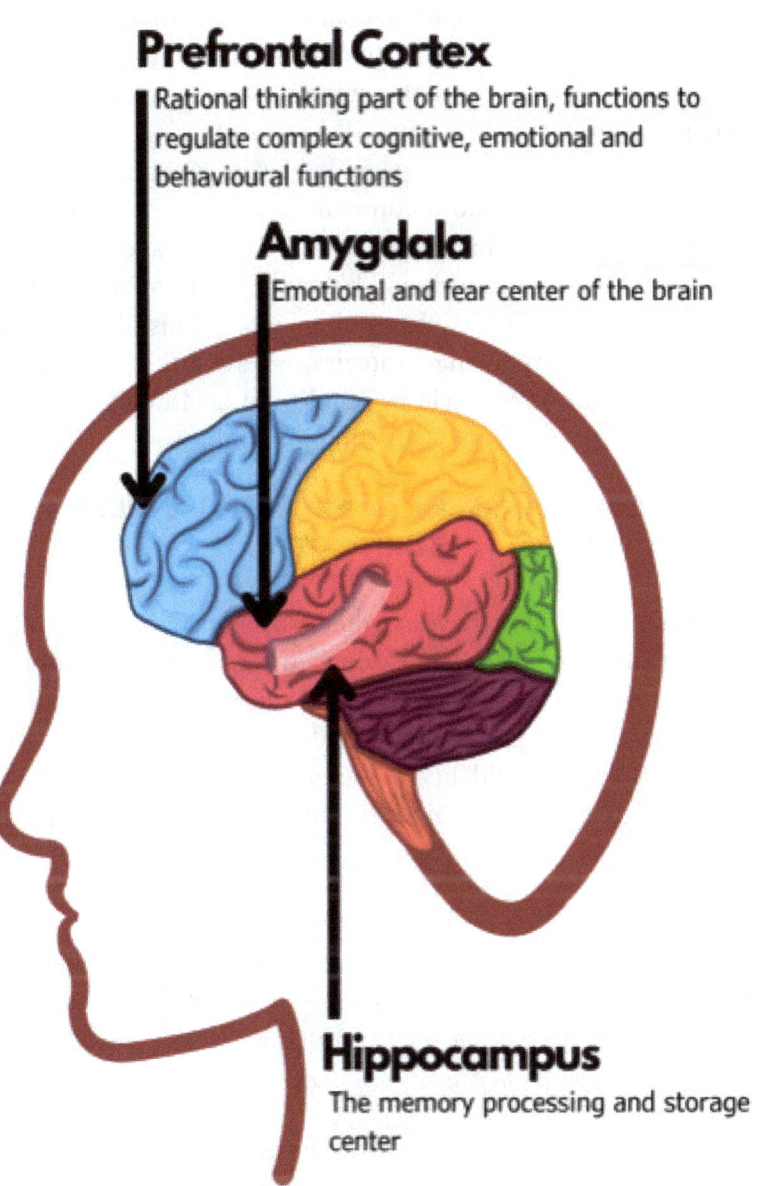

Figure 3: Brain showing the areas where stress and healing occur.

Uncontrollable stress and fatigue cause the release of inadequate or excessive levels of the chemicals that keep the brain alert (norepinephrine, dopamine, serotonin, acetylcholine) which cause the PFC brain (neural) connections to be lost, but restored when there is relief from the stressful situation. Additionally, with uncontrollable stress, the PFC gets thinner losing brain connections while the more primitive brain (amygdala) starts to get larger, and take a more dominant role. This, dysfunction of the PFC leads to the changes seen in the individual experiencing burnout;[22] like unprofessional behavior, lack of motivation, miscommunication with clients or patients. This also explains the role of stress-reducing strategies, whereby the individual is able to reset the stress cycle by employing healthy lifestyles like eating healthy, exercising, practicing mindfulness.

CONSEQUENCES OF EXCESSIVE STRESS (BURNOUT)

Certain professions have a higher risk for burnout, with studies showing that physicians are twice as the general population to experience burnout, depression[23] and suicide. And even among sub-specialties, it appears that family physicians have an even higher risk for suicidality.[23] Joiner Thomas' interpersonal-psychological theory explained why physicians commit suicide; whereby social alienation, perception of being a burden, and capability are factors.[24]

The consequences of burnout from chronic unattended stress are often grouped into[4]: *A. Extrinsic and B. Intrinsic outcomes; both further sub-divided into I) Physical and II) Psychosocial (which encompasses the emotional and behavioral) changes.*

Extrinsic consequences of burnout according to some researchers[15,4] include *i) reduced productivity arising from altered attentiveness and challenges with concentration from mental fogginess ii) reduced quality of care or service being provided, iii) decreased workforce, iv) increased absenteeism, v) decreased effective communication skills and* patient or client satisfaction, vi) more errors (medical and non-medical) , vii) early retirement or career switches and the resultant v) reduced mentoring opportunities.

Extrinsic psychosocial consequences include:[4] i) increased irritability ii) disruptiveness from being presented with higher tasks iii) decreased ability to empathize with clients or patients iv) strained worker-worker relationships but could be due to a person's personality and not strictly related to burnout.

Examples of **Intrinsic physical burnout outcomes** include i) severe exhaustion ii) increased cardiovascular disease like heart attacks from huge work demands with higher death rates[25], iii) higher motor vehicle accidents and work-related accidents (such as needle stick) with longer shifts (24hr vs. 16 as per Lemaire and Ghali),[26] iv) and deaths from accidental and non-accidental causes such as from suicide.

Other **intrinsic psychosocial consequences** include i) compassion fatigue, ii) moral distress and severe fatigue from witnessing patient sufferings, deaths, and day-to-day exposure to emotionally difficult situations[1], and iii) the inability to satisfy demanding patients/clients.[23]

Although not all agree, it is easy to see how stress and burnout influence substance abuse (e.g., excessive alcohol)[23] and medication overuse (sleep aids, pain relievers, muscle relaxants, anxiolytics) from attempting to treat the physical and psychological symptoms related to burnout. Other outcomes are strained relationships (e.g., separation, divorce), depression, substance abuse, suicide, strained marital and family relationships possibly from high work demand and non-protected time for relationships (boundary issues). Even without burnout, the rigor of medicine as a career[25] can negatively impact relationships. Some have reported high sickness-presenteeism in physicians linked to the culture of medicine.[23]

With the highlighted consequences found in physicians in mind, let's see how some other professionals' experiences are similar or dissimilar. My hypothesis is that compared with physicians, other professionals' burnout experiences will have a lot of intersectionality. And while the consequences may be similar, the burnout drivers will overlap in some areas and remain unique in others.

ANGIE THE SENIOR ADMINISTRATIVE SECRETARY

The other example I will share is that of an administrator at another big company in the city. This Caucasian female was playing a dual role including that of financial controller and senior executive administrative assistant for the company. Let's call her Angie. Angie has been in the company for over a decade already. In her case, her position has been static, given she has not risen through the ranks at all, but had salary increases only. The thing about her work was that she never truly had time off work on the weekends. Whenever her boss was travelling she and her phone were both on standby in case he needed anything.

Her workday started with yogurt -fruit parfait preparation for his snack because he told her it was part of her job. On the weekends, it was also her job to arrange taxis to-and-from the airport, book travel tickets in the event there was a flight disruption. Angie stayed late at work more days than not. It was easy for her to be taken advantage of partly because she was single and only had a dog she cared for at home. It would be straightforward, except that like everyone else she had her fair share of life throwing lemons at her every so often with her relative health taking a tumble!

Angie noticed that nothing she did was good enough. She felt compelled to work tirelessly to safeguard her job in the organization. Her mood began to suffer, exhaustion set in, sleep went south, and appetite swings which initially varied from day-to-day. She never stopped exercising mainly because she had a dog and could not bring herself to renege on her duty to it.

It seemed that the organization had grown bigger and began to hire more people, paying the new hires more for their services. A couple of the services were those she had provided in addition to her actual job description. It seemed unfair yet again. She was required to also provide training to the newcomers, and she was okay with that. The work environment appeared to be more gender diverse with a few more women hired into leadership roles. Angie is unable to tell which era was better than the other as they both came with their unique challenges. Although she did not have any interpersonal challenges with the male leaders, it seemed this was inevitable with the females.

Work began to be more challenging and the long years of service and hard work unrecognized by Angie's new leaders. She felt her work output was under-valued by the leadership, and couldn't but notice how her peers were getting promoted and not her. She surmised that the males were guaranteed a leadership position within a few years of being with the company, or so it seemed. She's spent over ten years already and is still at the same level, despite additional certifications and experience gathered on the job.

After many weeks of feeling desperate, confused, with lack of energy, Angie booked a medical appointment to see her family doctor. Her family doctor chose to prescribe time away from work and it has been several months yet. Her mood symptoms aligned with depression with some elements of anxiety such as irritability, worry about her future in the workplace and sleep difficulties.

Despite being off work, Angie shared that her boss insisted she kept the company's phone. This also meant that from time to time she still had to redirect customers to the right person who could assist them. Her phone continued to ring regularly for many months until recently.

Even though Angie knew to either temporarily return the work phone or power it off, she worried about losing her job while on sick leave or from 'pissing off' her new female Caucasian boss. *That's people-pleasing.* She also sacrificed her down time due to people-pleasing as it related to her former male Caucasian boss. The point in defining the race and gender of her bosses is to highlight the fact that gender and race might not always be at play, rather people's personalities and leadership styles.

CURTIS AND TRISH, THE ACCOUNTANTS

I initially considered focusing my book's target audience to professional women, until I met a young second-generation Caucasian male (parents were of European descent) on a plane recently. Curt seemed very caring and kind, not simply because he had assisted me with putting my hand luggage in the overhead bin, but from what I came to learn about his life and experiences. I didn't have to explain that my severely kinked neck muscle was the reason his help was needed before he gave it.

During our chat, I mentioned that I was writing a book on burnout titled *'Nothing Left to Give'* and was still undecided as to who my target audience was. His eyes sparkled and he proceeded to share his personal journey with burnout, and his partner's. Curt had no idea how much he contributed to confirming my initial thought about how common burnout was, sparing no one, regardless of gender.

He had gone into the accounting industry to please his parents as an only child. He never really wanted to go into the field, but the parental cultural expectation was such that children would either graduate from the university from one of three main fields: medicine, engineering, and accounting. I was surprised to hear about the similarity between the Ukrainian and Nigerian culture.

In general, people of Nigerian descent are not very different; in my days parents insisted that their children aim for medicine, law, or engineering in high school. Other courses were considered inferior, mostly based on limited exposure and narrow worldview of the vast opportunities that exist outside of the university and their preferred fields. However, people who gravitate into other fields or professions were less likely to be gainfully employed upon graduation from the university, due to the economy and limited marketability

Curt was willing to be vulnerable to a stranger and shared his experiences so freely. Though total strangers, we shared a connection – burnout. We exchanged phone numbers and decided to connect later. He promised to give me more burnout examples of male professionals he knew, some of whom had taken to maladaptive coping methods like excessive alcohol ingestion to help them sleep. He felt that my book's target audience could be expanded, and I agree. He mentioned that both he and Trish, his female partner (soon to be married), experienced burnout early on in their accounting profession. For Curt, his interactions with his immediate leaders varied irrespective of the genders assigned at birth. He did not feel that any one gender was necessarily better than the other in terms of showing compassion and empathy at the workplace.

His personal burnout trigger was mainly the high industry expectation that as an accountant one did not take time off during the tax season no matter what. One was seen as incompetent or weak, if they took needed rest from long hours poring over sheets of financial information required for income tax preparation. He shared how a good number of accountants, many of them males, resort to alcohol and other seemingly innocuous drugs as coping mechanisms which ultimately turns out to be a costly mistake in the long run.

He noticed his personality had changed; he was no longer looking forward to being at work because he was emotionally drained no matter what, despite applying sleep catch up periods. He hardly saw his partner and they were beginning to drift apart and the social connection with other family members and friends widening further. There didn't seem to be enough time in a twenty-four period to go to the movies or restaurant or do the other things they once loved. The interesting thing about Curt's situation was his partner was also experiencing similar symptoms with more relationship challenges.

He decided that he had to make a career change to cope. He felt less guilty switching careers because he had practically given his parents the gift they had wished for by becoming an accountant. He felt he could now do what he really wanted and felt no qualms about that. This decision led him into the mental health field where he became more aware about the barriers like the stigma, inadequate systems support associated with mental illness and their treatment.

Curt then made the tough decision to switch careers a second time. This time Curt felt drawn into policing, having availed himself of mental health resources with which he could make a positive impact in the society. He was all for being more compassionate, a factor needed in the Police Force and beyond. The plane ride we shared was to get him closer to his police force training. He would be spending about six months away from his partner, but I felt the palpable excitement about finally being in a career he was passionate about, doing something he had chosen himself. He felt he could incorporate *trauma-informed* or compassionate care as he went about his soon-to-be job.

His partner, on the other hand, did not make a career switch. She worked with her leader to improve the work culture and she is happier with the level of control she now has. She no longer had to drive to her workplace spending; or rather wasting precious time commuting over an hour each way because she lives in traffic-congested city in Ontario. She and her boss found a hybrid solution, something that was possible thanks to the pandemic which forced organizations and institutions to find alternatives to onsite work in physical office spaces from policies around social distancing. People initially switched to all virtual work and meeting spaces, and with time a combination of in-person and virtual options evolved.

ANDREW THE ENGINEER

During a mental health talk I gave at a church in Calgary, Andrew recognized some of the mental health changes that he experienced some years prior. He shared about his challenge in which he *'did not feel like himself, as though something was wrong'* with him. It seemed no one could understand him, and he began to withdraw into his shell and away from others the more. He also mentioned that he made good money, implying that money was not an issue for him at all. The issue wasn't Andrew's culture but work culture. For him, the burnout driver was the culture of perfectionism that gives no room for workers to bring their authentic selves into the workplace.

His story resonated with many as he described to the audience what he had experienced some years ago. Andrew's experience was not very dissimilar to some described already. Based on external appearances, the general assumption people held about him was that he was doing very well in every area of his life. Andrew has an African background, a professional in his field who was earning top dollars. Despite being financially stable, he had a hard time functioning the way he used to. His energy reserve had been depleted. He was living in a state of mental fogginess from day-to-day. He was able to go through the motion because he was familiar with the tasks to be handled each day. What he described seemed like using working memory as opposed to new ideas or creativity which was what he prided himself on. Andrew felt a disconnection from his loved ones as he grappled with the realization that 'nothing' gave him joy, neither his hobbies nor other social interactions with people in his social circle. He felt it was not worth the effort as he had little or no energy at the end or beginning of any given day. He panicked as he prayed he would not get any worse or live this way for the rest of his life. According to Andrew it took several visits to doctors before he finally deciphered what was wrong with him! He had also developed anxiety, fearing the worst. He thought something serious was wrong with him that was potentially deadly.

UNVEILING PERSONAL CULTURE: A DEEP DIVE

Sometimes it isn't work culture that is the issue, it is pressure we willingly take on that increases the chance that burnout results. Some professions like medicine have expectations that their workers will work over 60 to 80 hours a week, when administrative burden is added to the rigor of their day-to-day work. However, there are some cultural expectations in which members take on caregiving role and financial responsibility of immediate and extended family members. For some, this can be taken to very extreme heights whereby individuals take on two or more jobs to make ends meet. They work more than sixty hours a week for prolonged periods and in the process, neglect their own health, sacrificing rest and meaningful relationships.

Cultural expectations such as these can be a heavy burden for many. Some cultures expect that as soon as a family member leaves their countries of birth for greener pastures, the assumption is that money-trees have been planted in their backyards in advance of their arrival to the new country. In this fantasy, the individual just has to gather as much money from those trees as they wish, to send to their loved ones back home. This is an unrealistic expectation because it takes many months, if not years for people to settle and integrate into their new communities. Many of these individuals are truly resilient, but not putting boundaries early on can erode the fattest resilient bank account.

Other times it is the expectation individuals set on themselves that is partly the issue; yes, one's own drive for perfectionism through the eyes of other, *the Joneses*. The Joneses are other people who appear to have it all. The motive behind one's wants is hard to gauge, but one of the assumptions I am making is the need to have what the individual never had growing up.

In other words, it appears that experience with poverty and the compulsion to prevent it while noble, could be a burnout driver. The fear and anxiety of poverty have driven many to their graves early. The insatiable wants; the desire to be like others who don't give a hoot about one, the quest for riches and wealth to the point of sacrificing relationships is one such personal culture that increase the chance of experiencing burnout.

For some, owning designer brand items make them feel they have more value, and for others it is the posh cars and expensive homes with all the trimmings. There is nothing wrong with wanting the best for oneself, but to do so at a time and rate that is healthy would make more sense.

There is a time and season for the human body to perform at its peak, the years preceding middle-age. The adulthood phase offers a great opportunity to plan, making room for the rainy day. The other reality is that working extra hard for prolonged periods of time, increases the chance that the body will break down sooner than later, just as an unmaintained vehicle.

I find it quite disheartening hearing about early deaths of individuals that are often related to a lifestyle of neglect. Neglecting one's health is recipe for more troubles tomorrow, so imbibing a culture that invests in one's physical and mental health will go a longer way than one that attends to these areas much later in life. Investing in one's health includes preventative health and ensuring that one is up to date with screening for diseases and cancers that are preventable. Creating time for topping up on one's physical and mental health will lead to a life of happiness, good health and ability to enjoy life as independently as possible provided it is in our capacity. This is not intended to suggest that every person who is dependent on others for their activities of daily living was negligent of their physical or mental health. The key word is as much as is within one's control, living intentionally with health and wellbeing in mind would be rewarding, even if health challenges have already set in.

REFLECTION QUESTIONS

I suggest that you carry out the Reflection Questions before moving on to the next chapter because in each chapter are tips and ideas that would help you better understand the tasks ahead. Take your time and be sincere during your reflection of the following questions.

EXTRINSIC FACTORS: IDENTIFYING WORK-RELATED BURNOUT TRIGGERS.

Questions addressing Work-worker job mismatch

1. When was the last time you looked at your job contract?
2. What is your job title?
3. What are your role descriptions?
4. Does your organization's expectation of you align with what you are delivering from day to day?

Tip: Clarifying these will go a long way in preventing burnout. Yes, we can help in a time of need, but those moments should be in the short-term

Questions related to inadequate resources

1. Do you feel you are performing the job of two or more people?
2. Do you have the resources (equipment, training, mentoring, peer support) you need to perform a high-quality job? List the support you feel you need to succeed.

Questions addressing Work culture

1. What is your work culture like, e.g. a nurturing or toxic environment? Please give specific examples of why you feel this is the case.
2. How can the work culture be better, who can you turn to in order to achieve that?

3. Now, next question is what is within your locus of influence for effecting change in your work environment?

Questions addressing Organizational goals and values and worker wellness

1. What are your organization's values, mission, and vision?
2. Is worker health and wellness one of the priorities of your organization?
3. Do you have a wellness champion in your unit or division? What would it take to establish a culture of wellness in your organization or unit or division?

Tip: Sometimes it is easiest and best to start on a smaller and more manageable scale and then and then expand.

Questions addressing leader-worker dynamic and sense of belonging

1. Do you feel micromanaged or encouraged to make decisions with a reasonable amount of disapproval from your boss? Please list examples of times when you felt micromanaged or supported by your immediate leader?
2. What would you like to see happen? How can you achieve that- do you feel you can have that crucial conversation? Is there anyone within your organization you feel might be able to assist in having the crucial conversation? Why or Why not?

Questions addressing sense of inclusion and sense of belonging within the organization

1. Do you feel valued and appreciated by your organization and immediate leader?
2. How diverse is your organization? Do you feel a sense of inclusiveness and belonging in your organization?
3. Do you look forward to going to work on Monday, after the weekend? Why or why not?

4. Who can you go to for help in your organization (is there someone in the HR department you can reach out to for assistance in mitigating how things are going?
5. Have you already accessed the Human Resources (HR) department for assistance around your perception of feeling lack of belonging?
6. Did you find your experience with your organization's HR department helpful?

INTRINSIC FACTORS: THESE ARE PERSONAL FACTORS THAT MIGHT CONTRIBUTE TO BURNOUT

First, identify and write down what and who motivates you? This is an important step to finding out who you are and what makes you tick. It could open your eyes to some possibilities that have been dormant for a while.

Questions addressing organization-worker values mismatch.

Please reflect further and write down your own core values:

1. Do your core values align with that of your organization?
2. Questions addressing social connections.
3. Who forms your social support network?
4. Do you have an inner caucus within your social network, about two or three people you are comfortable being completely vulnerable with? For example, people who can give a good description of who you really are? This includes family members or friends from the community, church, or work?
5. What professional support do you have for yourself: This includes a financial advisor, spiritual leader, career coach, or therapist?

Questions addressing one's childhood and adulthood years and potential trauma

1. What was your childhood like? As far as you recall what was growing up in your home was like: *a) for you*, *b) through the eyes of your parents and c) how your parents interacted with each other?*
2. How about your relationship with your mom and dad (biological or foster parents) or the relatives who raised you? Were you an only child or had other sibling(s)? What was your relationship with your sibling(s) like?
3. As far as you recall, was there any childhood trauma? This includes bullying, poverty, loss of parent(s), significant others, accidents or other disasters?

Questions addressing financial stability and preparedness in case of disability or death

1. What are your finances like?
2. Have you had thoughts of your retirement? How close is retirement for you- in the horizon or do you still have a long time yet? What arrangements have you made for a comfortable retirement?
3. What would happen if you lost your job or had to walk out of your job tomorrow? Do you feel ready to make such a move? This question was posed to addresses one of the decisions that people have had to make when they feel they are unable to thrive within a toxic workplace any longer.
4. Have you ever thought of what would happen if the organization you have loved and come to call family should fold up tomorrow?
5. Although this is a difficult one, what plans have you made for your family and loved ones, in the event of your own or spouse's (or partner's if applicable) death?

Tip: If quitting your job means untold hardship for you and your loved ones, I suggest you ride it out until you have saved enough money for emergencies, or wait until you have another job offer, or are able to start your own business.

CHAPTER FOUR

FINDING YOUR HEALING

While burnout leads to severe consequences such that some feel like *'life is no longer worth living'* as they lose focus and sense of self-worth, it isn't supposed to take a person's life. It isn't a grave diagnosis like cancer or any other deadly disease. It can be managed through multi-pronged strategies. These will be discussed in the following chapters, please stay the course.

First and foremost, your personal holistic healing journey begins with system changes. Start by pressing on the brake pedal because the journey to wellness requires slowing down. Slowing down is the key to averting possible wreckage. Study after study has shown that there is no one method that is superior to the other, but approaches that are holistic in addressing burnout drivers are sure to go a longer way in not only managing it but preventing it.

Figure 4 provides suggestions for how to mitigate burnout at work level. Figure 5 is a schematic diagram depicting some holistic anti-burnout strategies[15] that support worker wellness.

A comprehensive approach[20] to mitigating burnout requires all levels involved to be evaluated and addressed. The burnout drivers will be listed followed by mitigating strategies. Although, this chapter mainly focuses on work-related strategies, there are Reflection Questions for the worker geared towards balancing work-life cycle.

CULTURAL CROSSROADS

i) Culture of Perfectionism tilted against worker realities

Organizations that are forward-thinking recognize that workplace errors are inevitable and proactively put structures and processes in place for mitigating them, be they human or equipment errors. For example, engaging in equipment maintenance culture has many benefits, like longevity, accuracy, efficiency and invariably higher quality output. Similarly, organizations with checks and balances in place for mitigating possible human errors has a better chance preventing them, and a lower chance of worse outcomes occurring.

Healthcare organizations can support high quality work among physicians and nurses by *encouraging learning* and being supportive of paid and unpaid continuing medical education to promote self-improvement. This makes workers feel that the system supports their career growth. The annual allocated amount for this learning need not be high.

A *review process for medical errors that balances grace and support for workers* allows workers to learn and grow from their mistakes. The use of heavy-handed (non-compassionate) approach can lead to stigma, shame, and other unintended consequences like anxiety, depression, or burnout. That said, the support for workers also needs to be balanced with client- or patient safety.

Another approach to mitigate errors is to *encourage workers to be collaborative* during processes and procedures. This reduces the chance that a surgeon operates on the wrong side of the body, if others participating in the surgical procedure are encouraged to assume some level of responsibility. The culture of *'sink or swim'* is not only toxic but is not nurturing.

Having a *buddy system* in place is another example of how to mitigate issues in the workplace. The worker, who is uncomfortable with any specific aspect of their work, should be encouraged to speak up and ask for support. Replacing the worker with someone else will only perpetuate a toxic culture. That worker could be supported with extra training or peer support for their areas of gaps or weakness. If we as humans are true to ourselves, we would admit that we are not strong in **ALL** areas.

The organization that creates room for authenticity is less likely to see an ongoing revolving door of workers quitting or moving on. It is true that humans will move on as they discover their passion and what motivates them, but their moves would be healthy and good for the organization. A workplace where quality and improvement are valued instils in workers the drive to go overboard, provided there is also some value placed on worker wellbeing. Workers that feel valued seek opportunities to make meaningful contributions in the workplace. Such worker might go beyond informal handovers to formal ones, by creating or updating standard operating manuals, and documenting the current status of key projects for their successors. This is a win-win situation for workers and organizations.

Systems and organizations may want to consider providing adequate training and support for the technologically challenged worker is worthwhile because of the resultant work efficiency that follows proficiency.

ii) Culture of Invincibility and 'Not Enough'

Sometimes organizations and systems drive high expectations of leaders and workers which in turn creates a culture that contributes to the sense of not being enough and invincibility. By balancing work expectations with worker capabilities whereby tasks they are passionate about are balanced with those that aren't necessarily their forte, the organization not only allows the worker to shine, but thrive through the support provided for areas of gaps. For instance providing a buddy system or supporting extra training as mitigation strategies could target such gaps.

Organizations could consider providing resources themselves or commit to providing a partial financial commitment to areas of worker interests that will in due course enhance and contribute to organizational strengths and excellence.

Policies that permit workers or workers to take needed time off when ill promote wellness. Investing in workers this way is likely to increase their sense of belonging to the point of being protective of the organization through a higher sense of accountability. Other than modeling, educating workers about the ills of sickness-presenteeism such as higher fatigue and errors is a wellness promoting strategy. Additionally, organizations need to walk the wellness talk by protecting worker break time and review shift duration from time to time. Reviewing shift duration alongside wellness conversations could be helpful in getting buy-in for modifying unpopular shifts so they are more manageable. This approach could be useful in reducing high sick call rates.

Adopting a balanced approach to scheduling, with backup plans for potential worker sick calls, and creating allowances on physician schedules for client or patient emergencies could be a useful tip.

iii) Work hour review

Oftentimes workers are hesitant about work hour modifications. As one can imagine, longer shift duration increases the risk of fatigue, errors, or difficult interpersonal relationships which also contribute to worker wellness concerns. Managers and senior leaders who recognize the issue and are keen to apply a different perspective to the issue are likely to have a higher chance of effecting change. The shift that no worker is keen to fill is another example of a work culture that requires change. With regular work hour reviews, leaders can address and modify shifts that appear to have a higher chance of being unfilled, and with higher absenteeism rates. From past experience, this suggestion might be unpopular with some workers without accompanying adjustments that negate income loss. In the long term, workers are better able to appreciate the need for prioritizing their wellness as it is closely linked with safer care, client and patient satisfaction and less room for errors.

iv) Culture of Diversity and Inclusion: Aiming for more than representation (inclusion)[1]

Promoting diversity without evidence of inclusiveness based on representation at all levels goes against the grain. Some describe it as an organizations' way of being able to tick off their checklist of having representation of diversity, which some have described as lip service. This speaks to the need for inclusion, where the diverse ideas and thoughts of the diverse groups are incorporated produces more comprehensive policies and programs, and offers better and more appealing solutions in the workplace. I commend organizations that have made significant progress in having a diversified workforce. Perhaps a next step would be finding similar representation at all levels; top to bottom. Policy and procedures revisions geared towards inclusivity, like inclusive hiring, remuneration, educational supports & grants supporting equity issues, leadership preparation, and mentoring opportunities are strategies to consider for mitigating non-inclusive policies, practices and procedures.

If there is no visible representation of minority groups at leadership level, then organizations need to go beyond 'tapping people on the shoulder', to a more active role in mentoring and training individuals from minority groups to be successful leaders. Another strategy might be supporting multi-stakeholder opportunities geared towards worker health and wellbeing, and other equity-advancing supports for minority groups.

v) Psychologically safe workplaces and conflict management

Toxic work environments, including *work COLA*; the culture of lack of authenticity, drives the lack of a sense of belonging and burnout at the workplace resulting in staffing issues from frequent work absenteeism and high turnover. Systems and organizations need to not only 'provide' a safe work place on paper, there needs to be clear processes for addressing worker-to-worker, worker-to-leader conflicts early. It could be useful to develop a clear path for leader-worker complaints processes (beyond the input of both the leader and worker) by a neutral body or team outside the local *Human Resources (HR)* department when there is conflict with a senior leader. Organizations insisting that workers address conflict through their immediate leader are contributing to the failure of the conflict resolution process. Firstly, the existing hierarchy between the leader and the worker creates a power imbalance and higher risk of worker punishment. Insisting on a single pathway for conflict resolution in such instances leaves the worker disenfranchised, hence fracturing the relationship further.

There are other times when workers might hesitate to involve their immediate leader when the worker-worker conflict indirectly involves that leader. For instance, if the worker for any reason feels that the leader and another worker have a close relationship; it could prevent them from going up to the leader to report any co-worker issues to the leader. An alternative approach to the worker who is choosing to bypass their immediate leader should be encouraged, whereby workers can reach out to HR to help resolve the worker's concerns. It could be that the third-party representation allows the worker to have the issue addressed early on. The HR staff's presence is to provide neutrality and objectivity to the conversations.

Established accountability processes that address specific toxic workplace behaviors and attitudes.

The utilization of clear processes for managing behaviors and attitudes that are toxic to the health and wellbeing of workers ought to be prioritized by systems and organizations. This involves using the same yardstick for addressing racism, discrimination, bullying and harassment, sexual and physical violence in the workplace. Ideally the process also includes the creation of a taskforce that includes an ombudsman highly versed in cultural sensitivity matters, in addition to anti-racist or other anti- inequity driven issues.

Policy changes are needed that foster inequity: Addressing the OQCE Roadblock Effect

Many immigrant professionals are interested mostly in their ability to provide food for their families and will often apply for jobs that they know they are overqualified for, since they are not readily accepted into their previous careers due to policy and procedures that serve as bottle neck. Many have assessed their circumstances and chosen to go with any available job to survive. They consistently face the OQCE roadblock which prevents them from being gainfully employed for many months, and years in some cases. This is especially true for immigrant professionals in the field of medicine, or engineering, and such.

OQCE phenomenon negatively impacts workplace diversity and contributes to disenfranchisement from pay inequities that arise from it, among others. Policies need to be provided for systems and organizations to assess individuals at the level they are applying. Not giving immigrants equal opportunity that allows them to be gainfully employed in their new country of residence goes so far as to fuel poverty, hardship, demoralization, higher mental health risks, heavier reliance on the system for social support to name a few. Provided immigrants have been accepted into the country, rules need to be relaxed around local experience. Their experiences in their country of birth or last residence should be used in determining their employability. Workplaces that parrot (no offense intended) *'you are overqualified, or you do not have Canadian experience,'* for instance, shut their doors to diversity, inclusion and equity. A better approach, beyond relaxing the rules around local experience is to provide additional support to ensure that people have the skills they claim to have, especially for fields where lives are not at risk. Health systems have processes for assessing readiness of practice for physicians, and the same model could be afforded other professionals as well.

Remuneration and Inequity issues: On the other end of the spectrum one can see from some of my clients' stories how being highly paid does not necessarily equate to worker satisfaction or wellness, rather the whole package of a good pay and a healthy work environment. What constitutes a healthy work environment is a balance of a sense of belonging from earning enough for work done as well as programs and initiatives that organizations provide that enhance worker growth, learning and their ability to thrive at the workplace. Making adequate allowances for worker remuneration, based on inflation and the like is forward thinking. It not only ensures that the worker feels adequately remunerated, they also can focus on getting their work done knowing that the organization will be looking after their needs.

Additionally, there is a need for ongoing fair remuneration review processes for the marginalized, under-represented, or non-unionized groups.

A CULTURE OF WELLNESS[27]

The drive for organizational excellence, without accompanying worker wellness focus, often creates problems. Systems and organizations come from a place of good intention, but utilizing top-down approaches for creating wellness programs and services have their issues. There are indeed times when a top-down approach is the most feasible or plausible approach to drive change. Nonetheless, without adequate checks and balances in place for the ongoing evaluation of progress and effectiveness of wellness programs, where changes or modifications are needed, they would not be readily evident. This approach could help address aspects of the issue of wellness initiatives at odds with work culture reality.

Other than ongoing evaluation of wellness programs, there is a need to invest in activities that support the promotion of workplace wellness culture. The best areas to focus on are those that are comprehensive and target major areas of need, which may or may not be self-identified by the workers themselves. For example, worker health programs should undergo ongoing review for possible need of expansion. Expansion of such programs should take into cognizance workers' feedback.

Another suggestion is refining organizational goals and values that include worker wellness and have a lead person to ensure alignment with the organizational goal of worker wellness. Yet another strategy is building coalitions with key multi-stakeholders with similar visions or goals.

Additionally, investing in worker appreciation and recognition could go a long way in increasing the sense of belonging and value that the worker feels. The best ways to show appreciation may need to be worker- identified at the unit or departmental level versus the senior executive level where worker appreciation may take the form of milestone recognition. For instance, a senior executive leader might want to send emails to workers who have spent five years, ten years, and the like. To add a gift with an organizational brand could be a good idea but might not resonate for all workers. It could be a good idea to have options for recognition for workers.

FOCUSING ON LEADERS[27]

Equip leaders to thrive

A focus on equipping leaders to succeed in their role goes a longer way in enhancing and improving workplace psychological safety and wellness. A leader who is equipped to perform well will impact many more in driving healthy workplace practices, for instance.

It goes without saying that ill-equipped leaders are at higher risk for fueling toxic work cultures through inability to adequately manage the handling of worker-to- worker, or leader-to-worker conflicts. The ill-equipped leader is also at higher risk to cause sanctuary trauma to co-workers. Similarly, organizations that do not have clearly outlined processes for handling psychologically unsafe worker behavior is one that is apt to run into problems sooner or later. The position of the organization needs to be clearly stated around anti-racist, discrimination, bullying or harassment behaviors in the workplace.

Leaders are humans and no one individual has it all. From hiring processes to leader orientation, the values of the organization need to be clear to the leader and other workers. By providing resources that point leaders and workers to educational materials around the organizational values, helps equip them and sets them up for success at the workplace.

For example, compassion, respect, avoidance of behaviors that perpetuate toxic work culture and environments and providing resources supporting learning and growth, wellness and conflict resolution strategies are a few ways to mitigate problems in this domain. Adequately equipped leaders are those who match gaps with learning opportunities e.g. cultural safety, *trauma-informed* approaches, conflict resolution, inclusive hiring practices. Both the organization and the leader have roles to play in narrowing any identified gaps.

Leaders are encouraged to find a useful leadership framework to help them perform better. For example, the **'LEADS framework'** which stands for Lead Self, Engage Others, Achieve Results, Develop Coalitions and System Transformation is one such that has been tried and tested. This was one of many other frameworks that I and others have found effective for leading change. I particularly like the *L (lead self)* portion because it promotes the practice of self-reflection as a leader. The leader who expects to be trusted must first demonstrate to others why they are dependable. It could also serve as a gauge in assessing one's emotion and behavior in the workplace, and possibly a reminder of the need to utilize a *trauma-informed* approach in all interactions.

360 degree Performance Reviews could be useful in encouraging self-reflection and mindfulness in leaders, with the realization that workers may be tapped to provide leader's feedback. Leaders are often assessed based on their ability to produce results or deliverables based on organizational goals.

Balance organizational -Worker expectations with current realities[15]

Another theme that contributed to burnout in the clients was reports of being assigned roles not defined by the worker's current job description. The issue here isn't that this cannot happen, rather that if they do occur, they should be few and far between, with the worker being relieved of one or more roles assigned to them on the day they have been tasked with training others for example. By *matching worker expectations with job descriptions* these frustrations can be mitigated.

Another example of imbalance in work-worker reality is one in which high worker expectation, isn't matched with adequate resources with which to perform those duties. Situations like this, are good only for promoting high staff turnover, more absenteeism, and higher burnout rates in their workers. High expectations of workers without adequate resources (e.g., human and equipment) contribute to delays in task completion and create highly stressful work environments and more conflicts in the workplace. Hence, *organizations need to invest time, energy, and money into providing adequate resources* to improve worker wellbeing in the workplace.

Balancing heavy reliance on technology: the use of online programs like electronic medical record (EMR) or electronic devices such as computers or iPads for completing work tasks are often cited as one of the reasons workers express frustration. The frustration comes in part from the occasional glitches that interfere with task execution and or completion. Systems that have a clear backup plan that workers can switch to avoid service disruption are better prepared to tackle the inevitable.

FOCUSING ON CLIENTS[27]

Moderating client expectations or demands.

High client expectations bring with it the potential for physical and verbal abuse toward workers, which can contribute to emotional exhaustion and burnout. So can the loopholes that create an imbalance between the drive for organizational excellence that is heavily client focused without adequately addressing workers wellbeing and increased sense of belonging.

Making posters visible and providing educational resources to clients or patients could be helpful in reducing the number of toxic interactions between workers and their clients. For instance, materials that clearly speak to the organizational value of providing a healthy workplace for their workers and clients, with an absolute zero tolerance for abuse, discrimination, racism, bullying, harassment, or violence upon registration. By providing pamphlets and forms with the stated psychologically safe and wellness values are likely to stimulate mindfulness on the part of both workers and clients. Having a back-up plan for handling physical or verbal aggression is important. Example, having an arrangement with security outfit, or not hesitating to call Emergency Protective Services when there are concerns of safety.

Another suggestion is investing in public systems that provide a guide on the procedures for balancing ideals with reality to help dispel shame, guilt, stigma, or trauma in the healthcare worker. For example, consider online protection for professionals at risk of suicide from harmful reviews.

While the earlier suggestions appear to be supportive of workers, ensuring a balanced review process for client or patient complaints is very important. The need to be patient-centered is important, with exceptions to this rule being instances when clients or patients are being abusive or displaying other forms of aggressive behaviors. There is a need to utilize a *trauma-informed* approach in ensuring that the worker is adequately cared for, and similar approach for resolving the conflict with the patient or client.

PERSONAL WORK-RELATED STRATEGIES

Personal work-related strategies that could mitigate burnout are approached in this section using accountability lens. There are two main accountability domains. That is, **accountability**

to self and ***to work*** (for example, colleagues, managers, or the organization).

Strategies for Enhancing Accountability to self:

- *Adopt healthy work practices such as prioritization work and boundary-setting. For example, prioritizing tasks and using work hours efficiently reduces the temptation to take work home. Secondly, equally important is adherence to boundaries around protected family time, except when work emergencies arise.*
- *Perform regular reflections on the quality and quantity of work done each day. Consider if there's anything else could have been done to make your work better each day.*
- *Identify gaps and seek learning opportunities to narrow those gaps. To do this effectively requires approaching this with authenticity.*
- *Practice gratitude, self-compassion, mindfulness, and other meditative exercises that make you a better person.*
- *Other wellness practices which start by allocating time for health and wellbeing through sustainable practices, some of which are avoiding diet fads, getting adequate sleep, picking up new hobbies and creating time for physical fitness. There are many more strategies that enhance your health and wellbeing that will be discussed in the next few chapters.*

Strategies for Enhancing Accountability to Others:

- *Watch for and acknowledge your biases and be careful they don't t show up in ways that are harmful to others.*
- *Practice kindness, compassion, openness, and flexibility, and be receptive to feedback in the workplace*
- *Advocacy: This can be through allyship for co-workers or managers who witness inappropriate and disrespectful behaviors in the workplace. For instance, consider speaking up against harmful practices to advance healthy work culture and wellbeing. Consider ways, if any, of sharing one's power and privilege with minority groups. Many have said that 'not speaking up' could be interpreted as condoning injustice and inadvertently gives perpetrators more*

power to continue with harmful behaviors.
- *Build strong social work connections because this allows you to learn from others and to share your work with them too.*

SYSTEM STRATEGIES

CULTURAL
- Promote cultures that balance reality with expectations
- Balance client focus with worker sense worth

INNOVATION & CREATIVITY
- Adopt objective measurement tools and continuously adapt
- Utilize comprehensive approaches to issues by mixing-matching, collaboration

POLITICS & POLICIES
- Policy and procedures geared towards equity
- Adopt collaborative processes and close loops during re-structuring
- Promote Equity, Diversity and Inclusion: hiring practices, retention, grants and other educational supports

REMUNERATION ISSUES
- Regularly review payment scales in the face of inflation
- Create room for payment review of marginalized underrepresented and non-unionized workers

ORGANIZATIONAL STRATEGIES

CULTURAL
- Adopt inclusive cultures: 'everyone together' approaches encourage worker authenticity by practicing what you preach, encourage worker self-agency

HEALTHY WORK ENVIRONMENT TIPS
- Educational Supports
- Workplace Ergonomics
- Mentoring and Peer Support opportunities
- Establish specific tribunal or ombudsmen for anti-racism and other psychologically unsafe behaviors Program Support
- Support accountability and establish anti-racist and anti-discriminatory policies and procedures
- Promote worker appreciation and sense of value: peer-to-peer, leader-worker activities

MATCHING WORK-WORKER EXPECTATIONS
- Align leadership roles with decision-making authority for meaningfulness
- Match work-worker roles and responsibilities based on job contract

LEADERSHIP ISSUES
- Balance autocratic-collaborative leadership styles
- Equipped leaders with tools needed to thrive in their roles
- Adapt Worker Periodic Review processes to be holistic and multi-faceted for assessing performance
- Communication issues: balance frequency with effective communication

PERSONAL STRATEGIES

- Accountability
  - To Self
  - To Work
- Adopt healthy work practices including boundary-setting
- Perform own reflection on quality and quantity of work done
- Identify own gaps and seek learning opportunities to narrow those gaps
- Avoid the temptation to take work home:
  - Set time for work
  - Prioritization
  - Boundary-setting

Figure 4: Work-related Burnout Mitigating Strategy

REFLECTION QUESTIONS

QUESTIONS FOR WORKERS

Below are some examples of questions to try and ponder over as a way of finding solutions that will likely be helpful for your unique work setting.

1. What is culture in the environment where you work? For example, is it supportive, collaborative, toxic or unwelcoming? Has it always been this way? What changed and when?
2. What type of dynamic do you have with your colleagues, immediate leader, higher level leadership?
3. How would others describe your attitude to work, e.g. perfectionist (you find it hard to delegate tasks to others because you don't trust that they will do a perfect job), workaholic (you work tirelessly and when work out to be done, you continue to prioritize work over family time) , people-pleasing (you go out of your way to please people, even when you don't have the capacity)?
4. How would others describe your personality: extrovert (very outgoing, friendly, not shy), introvert (you like to play it safe with strangers, you are reserved) , or a hybrid (can socialize with strangers in some settings or specific situations?
5. How would you describe yourself in terms of preference for getting work done— *collaborative, solo approach or hybrid?*
6. Do you feel psychologically safe at work?
7. Do you feel a sense of belonging (whereby you feel that your thoughts and ideas are valued and incorporated when decisions are being made) in the organization? Why? Why not?

If you feel strongly about advocating for change at higher levels, the following questions are for you to consider:

1. Do you feel valued by the overall system or industry—why or why not?
2. What would you like to see happen at higher industry levels? What have you done personally to advance what you think are noble and worthy causes to improve the industry? What is holding you back? Who do you need to connect with to start the process (for example, mayors?)
3. Who else is passionate about making a positive change in your work environment or in the community?
4. Have you considered a multi-nodal (multi-pronged) approach to system change (that is, you have assessed the different areas that require improvement, and also considered the various key stakeholders with interest in the area)? What would that look like for you?

QUESTIONS FOR LEADERS

1. What are your organization's values?
2. Do your values include diversity and inclusiveness and worker wellness? Yes or no, and, why or why not?
3. How diverse is your current work environment? Is there equal representation across the board, from top to bottom? That is, by what percentage are there workers with diverse and ethnic minority backgrounds? Do you have a similar percentage represented in upper management positions? If not, why, or why not?
4. How important is worker wellbeing to your organization on a scale of 1-10? If the rating is less than 8, why is that the case?
5. In what ways are you and or your organization supporting worker wellbeing? How is that working out? Have you been able to assess the effectiveness of your current wellness initiatives? Why or why not-what are the pros and cons? What would it take to evaluate the wellness initiatives you have?

6. What method(s) do you utilize for performance reviews? Do you use the same indicators for workers as for leaders? Is it 360 degrees- meaning peers, immediate leaders and other allied colleagues? What areas of leadership do you assess? Do these include conflict management, cultural and psychologically safe aspects? Do you encourage leaders to self-identify gaps or areas of challenges that need support?
7. How would you describe your leadership style, for example, autocratic or collaborative or *trauma-informed*? Have you had to adapt your leadership style in the last year or two? How so? What brought about the need for change?
8. What do others say of your leadership style?
9. Do you feel equipped to lead? *Yes or No?* How confident are you managing human resource issues? How about effectively managing worker-worker conflicts? What are the barriers or challenges you face during worker interactions?

CHAPTER FIVE

THE MIRACLE OF GETTING AWAY

Adopting a holistic approach to health and well-being, that combine system and personal level strategies[27] is the best way to prevent and manage burnout. Having addressed work-related strategies in previous chapters, the rest of this book focuses on personal strategies for healing from and preventing burnout. See Figure 5 for some examples. This chapter uses the analogy of getting away to mean *away from everything that constitutes stress;* those steps that allows one look inward. In other words, getting away from distractions through various mindfulness-based exercises, or physically stepping away from work or the home environment allows the mind and body to reset.

THE WELLNESS-RESILIENCE FACTOR

The false assumption that only weak people experience burnout only perpetuates stigma, and many people often think that with regards to resilience, one *either has it or not*. This couldn't be further from the truth! Resilience is not a static factor and in this section, we will explore resilience from a different perspective—one that invalidates this misconception and fosters healing.

It is important to access your resilience level to determine the appropriate coping strategies that target the specific burnout level you are experiencing (mild, moderate, or severe.) According to Brené Brown, resilience can be looked at from three perspectives, *i) personalization in which individuals believe they are the problem, ii) permanence arising from cognitive distortions that suggest that the challenging situation is here to stay creating more stress and anxiety, and lastly iii) pervasiveness which contributes to the feeling of despair and despondency where hope becomes quite blurry and 'nothing good is left'*[13]. The further down the burnout scale you find yourself, the higher the despair level and the lower the resilience level.

Achieving wellness and preventing burnout requires an assessment of your wellness-resilience bank account.[28] This means taking stock of where you are on the wellness-resilience scale and assessing where you would like to be in the future. In this process, you must take the time to identify gaps in your wellness-resilience journey and begin practicing strategies to narrow those gaps. Dr. Michael Maddeus, a thoracic surgeon, discusses the importance of the resilience bank account. Since the purpose of the resilience bank account is to make rich deposits aimed at wellness, I am choosing to call it the *wellness-resilience bank account*.

The process starts with *self-acceptance* and *self-compassion*. Embrace yourself—beauty and flaws inclusive—and be kind to yourself. A person with lower wellness-resilience bank account has a higher chance of being burned out and burnout happens to the best of us, regardless of how well stocked our account was initially. Unless you practice constant renewal of your wellness-resilience bank account, your chance of burnout rises higher as the account starts depleting.

The wellness-resilience bank account will grow as soon as you start investing in healthy wellness practices that promote resilience. The fatter your wellness-resilience bank account is, the more withdrawals you person can make without going into a deficit. A few ways to make those deposits are ensuring one gets adequate sleep, eats healthy diet, exercises, and purposefully practices like self-compassion, meditation, and gratitude.

Others are boundary-setting—saying **NO** in a respectful manner when your plate is too full and following through— and creating time to give back to the community through acts of volunteerism are other examples of resilience deposits.

The rest of the chapter and the rest of the book build upon strategies that have been meaningful and effective for burnout prevention and healing.

THE PRACTICE OF MINDFULNESS AND MEDITATION[23]

Mindfulness is an ancient practice. Though, it is practiced with various variations and methods, it is all aimed towards encouraging individuals to be in the present while being nonjudgmental of any negative feelings that arise.[16] This state of mind has been described as *'being in the zone, going with the flow, with meditation in action describing a state in which the individual is constantly identifying their thoughts, feelings and emotions shift throughout the day'*[29] The benefits of mindfulness cannot be overemphasized, as it improves one's ability to concentrate, lowers stress level, connect meaningfully with colleagues, improves productivity and prepares one to anticipate events before they occur.

Examples of mindfulness include[16]:

- *Body scan: in which you notice bodily sensations and the cognitive and emotional reactions associated with those sensations without an attempt to change the sensations;*
- *Sitting meditation: involves silent meditation in a seated position*

> that brings awareness to thoughts, feelings, and sensations experienced in the moment;
> - *Walking meditation: brings awareness to the experience of slow, deliberate, and attentive walking; and*
> - *Mindful movement: this includes yoga-type exercises done in a way that allows the exploration of the sensory, emotional, and cognitive aspects of the experience.*

Tarthang Tulku cited by Davich[30] said *'Caring about our work, liking, or even loving it might seem strange only when work is seen as a way to make a living. But when work is seen as an opportunity to deepen and enrich our experiences, one can find caring in one's heart, awaken it in others as one uses work to learn and grow'.*

Meditation in action helps me reset my stress button more often than waiting to do the Reflective Practice at the end of each workday would. Meditation in action allows one to not carry negative energy with them into other spaces.

SELF-AWARENESS, FORGIVENESS AND SELF-COMPASSION

Reflecting on your core values, evaluating and correcting any misalignment of your priorities and those of your significant others is a self-awareness practice that is beneficial to healing. Self-awareness is the important first step to healing and resetting the mind and body. Be aware that self-awareness could trigger self-loathing or guilt over mistakes of the past, so it should be paired with self-compassion.

Let go of the past. Letting go is crucial to moving forward in your healing journey. Forgiveness starts with you and me. We must forgive ourselves first, or we will likely have difficulty forgiving others; this is an essential aspect of self-compassion. The other aspect is that of being kind to self as to others. Forgiveness does not mean forgetting about negative experiences. It means *choosing to let go of the hurt, not because the other person deserves it.*

I once had a client with significant childhood trauma share her recent attitude to her past hurts and anxiety about the future. The hurt that impacted her self-confidence at work. She said *'I only dwell on the positive aspects of the past where I felt love and stay in the moment much longer, with very brief visits to the future.' By approaching life this way, this client has begun to enjoy li*fe in a way that she hadn't for some decades. This was key in her ability to forgive those who hurt her and defining the terms of ongoing relationship. She replaced the anger she felt with empathy. The practice of letting go of past hurts is important for the success of any relationship, personal or professional.

I find that letting go of past hurt allows me to approach each moment and each day with a full tank. The past stands in my way of sleep and is an impediment to one's progress at home, work or community. This is because past hurts stand in the way of striking new friendships because everything and everyone is assessed not on their own merit rather from pre-determined yardsticks created by others.

Several Bible passages that speak about the need to forgive others as many times as possible, to process anger or hurt in healthy ways and to let them go. For instance, the book of *Ephesians 4:26* states that *'when you are angry, do not sin, do not let the sun go down while you are still angry'*. Listening to people's stories, I find there is often fear and anxiety around forgiveness. It appears forgiveness is thought to equal erasure of the negative experiences as though they did not occur. To do so would be to hinder one's healing. The brain is wired to heal, and not processing negative experiences can lead to 'being stuck' since the brain has not been given the opportunity to heal from those negative experiences.

Being able to forgive and set boundaries is one of many approaches to not letting the past define me.

THE POWER OF PAUSE

My personal burnout prevention recipe need not be yours; mine will likely be different than yours, with a few similarities. To heal adequately from burnout, I began to make time for travel, spa days, community connections, leadership, philanthropy, and continue to eat healthy diet and regularly exercise on most days. My burnout prevention recipe also includes managing my finances and learning to say no to requests for my time that don't align with my values. To be honest, saying NO is the most difficult coping strategy for me as it might for some others. I am still working on that, and many other boundary issues.

Taking some **time off work and medical training** during the period of burnout was crucial to replenishment following the realization that I was depleted. As a resident physician, taking leave of absence meant time away from the learning environment and the need to extend the training by the equivalent amount of time. I chose to focus on my renewal than worry about the latter. This also required correcting the brain's cognitive distorted thoughts of invincibility to burnout or any other health problems. With the practice of mindfulness, the concept of sickness-presenteeism was dealt with. This meant that learning to **be present** whenever I showed up, whether it was in a learning or work environment. 'Be present' has become one of a few mantras.

The worry about financial situation[31] often leads to working excessively which is often an overcompensation that could be detrimental to people's health. For example, working two jobs or longer hours to meet up with a financial need, often derails healthy lifestyle. It is easy to see how sleep deprivation, no time or energy to exercise, cook healthy meals or maintain healthy social connections. The trouble with this way of thinking is that it does not take into full consideration that with time, the uncared-for body will break down, regardless of one's financial status at the time. Granted everyone's situation is different and not many can afford to take the needed time off work, especially when if self-employed due to the many financial obligations. *Not creating time to rest is synonymous to continuing to drive a car needing maintenance.*

First, I had to deal with the anxiety that came from the possibility of extending my training because I took a stress leave. Thankfully, after my program director reviewed my assessment, that period of absence was waived, much to my excitement. The waiver of the training extension was the icing on the cake to being renewed from taking time off.

The importance of taking a step back for anyone with signs and symptoms of burnout cannot be overemphasized. This can happen in various ways—from modifying your work schedule to shorter days, taking weekends off, or scheduling regular short or even long breaks. You know what might work best for your unique situation and needs. That said, sometimes people are unaware of how much time off they might need to reset, because they fail to realize that they are burned out before others start cluing in. Hence, my suggestion is to take more time than you think you might need. For example, plan to take two weeks off if you can, even if you think one week would be sufficient. Alternatively, a health and wellness professional such as mental health therapist and or family physician might be able to assist in determining the length of time needed, depending on the severity.

THE POWER OF SLEEP[32]

By discussing the importance of sleep to reset our body and mind early on, is a reminder of its importance. To make time for this seemingly passive activity each day, is to prevent burnout and aid faster healing. Sleep deprivation is a major contributor to motor vehicle accidents, burnout, anxiety and depression, and other health issues like diabetes, especially when it becomes a chronic issue. Chronic sleep disruption alters the body's natural circadian rhythm which in turn leads to consequences like burnout, errors, and involuntary sleep attacks called microsleeps that are often implicated in motor vehicle accidents, and a decline in working memory. The body's altered ability to produce adequate levels of melatonin causes insomnia and insulin resistance which is contributes to the development of Type 2 Diabetes.

Sleep is a top priority for wellness and burnout prevention. The power of sleep to rejuvenate cannot be overstated. To have adequate sleep, ideally one needs to rest for about 7-9 hours overnight. Although the school of thought is that individuals require 5 hours of sleep to be cognitively alert, the recommendation is 7-9 hours overnight. It is during sleep that our brain gets to turn off, the muscles and the rest of the body relaxes.

There are many useful tips on getting adequate sleep, such as keeping a regular sleep schedule, avoiding stimulating activities like exercising close to bedtime, reducing caffeinated beverages, and avoiding them after 2 p.m. in the afternoon since their effects can last several hours later, ensuring the bedroom is used for sleep and intimacy only; and avoid watching T.V. or utilizing other electronic devices. Other sleep hygiene tips include setting aside some time to prepare for bedtime routines like showering, brushing one's teeth and other activities that help set the stage for sound sleep, creating time to catch up on sleep deficits during the weekends, or power napping for about ten to fifteen minutes during the day.

Napping in the daytime is not something my body is used to. I'm always amazed when people say that they feel refreshed to tackle the rest of the day after merely taking *a power nap* during lunch break. Sleep remains an area needing work after over a decade of being 'on call'. I had to find alternative paths to solving my sleep issue. My issue is not initiating sleep, but maintaining sleep. By default, I go to bed only when I am tired. Somehow, my sleep clock has been set to wake up at about four in the morning, regardless of when I go to bed. With my family doctor's input, mild-to-moderate sedatives were tried, but side effects were limiting. The specific side effects: grogginess, difficulty focusing or get any meaningful work done for a couple of days at the smallest dose.

Hence, the more natural way of treating insomnia that worked for me was mindfulness practice (which I will describe briefly below) if I am having a challenge initiating sleep. At other times, simply drinking warm non-caffeinated beverage, having a warm shower, and ensuring the room temperature isn't too cold or too hot, are some tips that have been quite useful to manage my sleep disturbance. Below is a description of progressive muscular relaxation which was useful in addressing the challenge of sleep initiation.

SLEEP INDUCTION: PROGRESSIVE MUSCULAR RELAXATION.

This practice of the art of mindfulness involves simultaneously tensing and relaxing various muscle groups starting from the toes, progressing to the trunk, the hands arms and head and neck and head and facial region. It has been a helpful practice for resolving trouble initiating sleep some nights.

THE WISDOM OF WANDERLUST

In this chapter, I will share with you why travel is such a vital part of preventing burnout and a highly effective way to recover from burnout. Travel looks different for everyone. We all love to travel differently. Some love luxurious travel and some prefer camping or backpacking. The key to utilizing travel to benefit your mental health and add to your wellness-resilience bank account is that it forces one to pause, step away from the mundane and work, and in most cases rest from household chores and unending errands!

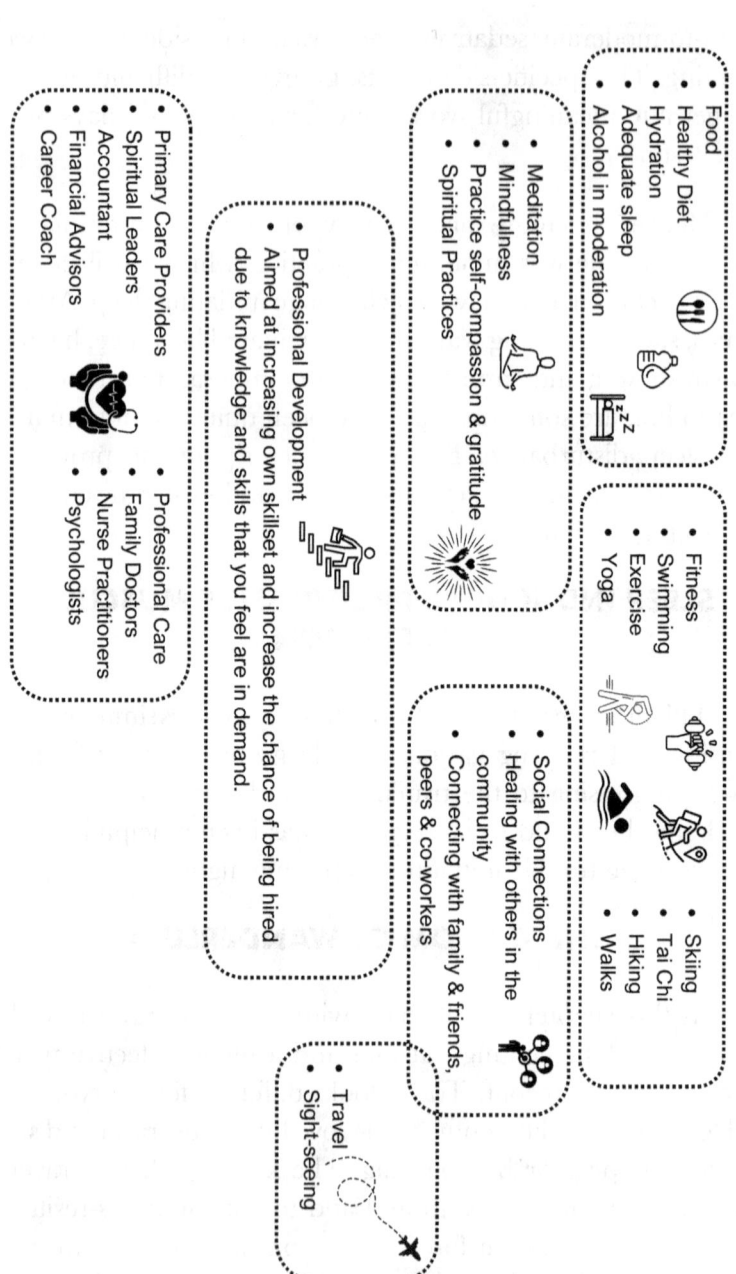

Figure 5: Personal Burnout mitigating strategies

In 2010 when I first experienced burnout, I travelled to Nigeria after about five years of being away from my country of birth. I had lost significant amount of weight around this time and I was two dress sizes down. I was not trying to lose weight; things had fallen apart at the home-front just as I was wrapping up my residency training.

The trip to Nigeria helped me reset faster than any antidepressant could. Earlier, I mentioned that antidepressants were prescribed to help me with what appeared to be an adjustment reaction. And in the course of the treatment, I found out that my body was very sensitive to medications, which led to settling for one called Wellbutrin which I tolerated for a little longer than the others. Seeing my siblings and other family members helped me reset quite quickly. I was treated to local delicacies and the humid weather felt good for my skin and hair. I did not appreciate the heat though, but there is always a way around that - many people have generators in their homes because electricity was not constant. However, the food is freshly made with organic vegetables and all the other condiments. The dishes are mouth-watering. Despite the temptation to eat every dish put in front of me, eating sensibly during trips like this is something I'm mindful of. My go to being protein, vegetables and fruits over foods high in saturated fats and refined carbohydrates.

Going from city to city, by road or by air to visit with friends and family members is sometimes not convenient. Hoever, the cultural expectation is such that people would take offense if one did not visit them, even if one's trip was short. Usually, I go with gifts and money for friends and family, and like our culture expects, they would host me and feed me well.

The main reason for travelling was to de-stress. I felt the need to clear my head, and was successful at that during the two-week period that I spent in Nigeria. For me, leaving Calgary, Canada away from work and other stressful situations allows me to sleep, not troubleshoot as much, eat well and rest. It is during such trips that I appreciate the nature around me, the food, and the people much more. So, at the end of this trip there was clarity of mind which was what I had hoped for. Beyond material things, I needed peace like never before. Living a peaceful life would take me back to where I always was as a young adult.

My love for travel began at an early age. Almost every weekend dad made sure to take the whole family to our hometown or a neighboring city or the other. Those were fun childhood days as it meant we could literally roam around the town and go to places we would otherwise not visit. For example, whenever we visited our hometown in Eastern Nigeria, we would sneak out to the riverside even though we did not actually know how to swim. The way to the river was sort of an Eco Trek. We usually went in larger numbers; about six to eight of us siblings and a few relatives. We would stop every now and then to pick fruits from fruit trees.

We loved stopping at relatives' houses along our way unannounced, especially if it was during festive seasons like Easter or Christmas. Sometimes our parents would be entertaining guests and hardly noticed we were out for what we called our 'freedom' hike trusting our relatives who were about the same ages as us to guide us.

FEARFUL SKIES

From the moment I was able to afford traveling with my kids, the decision made was ensuring we visited different cities or countries each year. Our first intentional trip to de-stress was to Cancun, Mexico. The biggest draw to Cancun was the fact that there were several options for an all-inclusive resort trip, with lots of restaurant options, family-friendly activities, plus a break from work and school runs, and household chores. It was great to not have to wake up early and be able to take in the beauty of the place. Besides eating and sleeping in, we also limited our walks to the resort area, unless we were going on a group tour.

We were all excited. We all fell in love with our ocean view suite from where I could appreciate the expanse of the ocean and the sky meeting, the further away one looked. It was exhilarating and felt natural to relax and unwind. This trip provided a happy space after a long time of too much work. I began to write again on this trip, after over a decade of putting it in the back burner since arriving in Canada. Other than practicing being in the moment where I noticed the beauty around me, there was also a sudden urge to write again. It wasn't anything complicated, just using Cancun as an acronym to reflect how I was feeling.

Honestly, I don't know what sparked my creativity. I wonder if it had anything to do with the environment, the ocean view and large expanse of beach on the property. Below is what I came up with from my self-reflection:

Flying across the globe, thousands of miles away with three kids in tow, clueless as to what to expect on this trip to C-A-N-C-U-N, the uncertainty sparking my curiosity and creativity:

C: Clarity; fogginess cleared
A: Appreciative of life, my very many blessings
N: Novelty; newness of mind
C: Concentrating on the things that matter
U: Uncluttered, letting go of the past
N: New birth, new beginning for today an attempt is made to write again

We explored many places in Cancun, taking photos with the dolphins and beautiful architecture. The array of Mexican dishes like tacos, fried beans, and rice dishes were truly sumptuous. The tropical fruits were the highlight— mangoes, pineapple, papaya, avocados. It was nostalgic for me, reminding me of my childhood.

Talking about new discoveries from the Cancun trip, other than the serenity of the place and the fun activities, we noticed something else. No one had bargained or prepared for the discovery of a phobia for flying in one of my kids! So, I needed to reassure my seven-year-old that he would be fine. It took many more plane rides and arranging which kid sat next to me on the plane before he became comfortable flying. Luckily, Cancun was wonderful trip for all three of us regardless of the stress of flying related to the phobia for flying.

When we visited Puerto Vallarta, Mexico, we learned to snorkel. Despite being novices at best, it was an amazing experience to see life underwater!

Our Caribbean adventures saw us in Dominican Republic, San Juan, Puerto Rico, Barbados, St. Georges, Grenada, Roseau, Dominica, St. Philipsburg, St. Maarten, and Tortola in British Virgin Islands. We witnessed their communal ways of life that resembles those of many African cultures.

We also visited a number of places in the United States like the San Diego Zoo in California, LEGOLAND, Disney World, and Empire State building in New York. Some of these trips were during medical conferences so I combine learning with adventure. As of now, I've been to twenty-seven countries, including Florence in Italy, Spain, Japan, South Korea and the United Arab Emirates.

Our Canadian getaways have been limited probably because of the perception that they are right at the fingertips. Nonetheless, Montreal City, Niagara Falls, Saskatoon, Vancouver, Greater Toronto Area, with stops at China Town, Marine Land, Eaton Centre, and Winnipeg are other cities we have visited or lived in while transitioning from Toronto. Other tourist areas worth visiting include Canmore and Banff which are in the province of Alberta—they are known for the breath-taking mountain-views worth visiting as a get-away from the busyness of the city. If one enjoys soaking their muscles in hot tubs, Banff Hot Springs could be a good stop while in Banff, especially during the winter season. It is an amazing experience, despite the outside minus-degree temperature.

In Banff, we camped outdoors with a church group. Although we were wary of bears, we enjoyed the traditional camping experience whereby we put up a tent with help from the friends from church, laid on mattresses placed on taupe with bedding and lots of blankets to keep warm overnight as temperatures typically fall overnight, and used the campsite bathrooms and toilets for bio breaks. We cooked light meals over firewood that tasted very good, flavored by the smoke. It didn't matter that it was fried eggs, bacon and pancakes, all the while mindful not to leave food out, to avoid attracting bears. Yes, Banff is a *'Bear Country'*.

With the church group we met up with, we participated in various activities including hiking around the area. Perhaps my next camping experience will be non-traditional; in a cozier lodge camper where I would have a better night's sleep and worry less about a bear sniffing around the tent. Exploring the Canadian East Coast is climbing up my travel list.

To conclude, travel isn't just about seeing the world. It's about discovering new passions, hobbies, friends, and who you truly are. If you don't enjoy travelling or feel it is out of your reach, keep reading as there's more tips for wellness and burnout prevention to come!

REFLECTION QUESTIONS

1. What is your mantra, if any? If you don't have any, can you take some time to write down your new mantra? Doing so will help you regain focus when your practices begin to slip, so I encourage you to try writing one down.
2. What areas of healthy lifestyle practices, might you be struggling with the most? Which ones are easier?
3. Do you love travelling out of town or simply getting away for the weekend? How has travel been good for your soul?
4. What has travel taught you about other people's cultures, their foods and languages?
5. What is the earliest travel experience you can remember? Did it create a love for traveling?
6. If you have children, nieces or nephews, have you taken the time to expose them to nature around the community where you live, or travel (locally or internationally) thereby broadening their world views?

CHAPTER SIX

THE BODY'S ABILITY TO HEAL THROUGH FITNESS AND FOOD

HEALING THROUGH FITNESS[23,27]

Stress always manifests in our bodies. It is the body's job to communicate to our brain when something is wrong or needs to change in our lives. For this reason, it is imperative that we care for the body. The role of exercise in maintaining physical and mental health is well-established. *Canada Fitness Guide* recommends one hundred and fifty minutes a week of exercise.[33]

During exercise, the brain releases endorphins which are *'happy'* chemicals. Exercise increases a person's ability to focus and does prevent and helps to manage diseases such as arthritis, fibromyalgia, hypertension, diabetes, obesity, and depression. Although exercise helps to prevent and manage burnout, on its own, it is insufficient as a singular personal coping strategy.

The recommended amount of exercise is less than three hours a week, and the beauty of this is that it can be tailored individually. For instance, one could exercise every other day for thirty to forty-five minutes, or an hour on one day and the rest on another or cram them up weekly. I do not recommend the latter because overworked muscles are painful muscles and painful muscles reduce the chance of creating a consistent exercise practice.

Combining activities that increase one's heart rate with stretching and strengthening is the way to go. Walking leisurely to start, interspersing that with intermittent brisk walking leads to a similar result as jogging, provided the duration is extended. The goal is to increase one's heart rate during any chosen activity and to maintain it for as long as possible to break down calories.

In this chapter I share some of my experiences with different types of fitness activities. My goal is to encourage you to be flexible, get curious about new fitness activities, try them, and then select what works best for you.

NATURE'S THERAPY

Fitness for the purpose of staying healthy is something I learned on my own. Neither of my parents were athletic, but they did ensure they ate healthy meals and avoided excessive intake of salt and sugar. They purchased bikes for us, but did not necessarily state that we were to ride our bikes every day and for an hour, or anything like that. We just did. My siblings and I almost always went for long walks with our neighborhood kids. We went in groups, and no one asked the specifics of where we were headed. I guess the assumption that *'there's safety in numbers'* was established around this time. Unknown to our parents, sometimes these were long walks to the nearby river, even though we did not know how to swim! Other times we simply rode our bikes.

As far as physical activity goes for me in Canada, my hosts (way back when) owned an eight-year-old German shepherd,

Max, that I came to love. I loved Max because upon my arrival at the house he sniffed me and that was it. We became buddies. There were also two other Dalmatian dogs that my hosts' son owned. Those two were full of energy and when they were not yapping, they licked everything within their reach.

My hosts walked their dog daily and soon I was doing the same. The dog would wake me up early in the morning around 6.30am and I would take it out to go do its business outside the property. Growing up, we didn't really have to walk Roger, our dog. It walked around the house and had a very long leash when we needed to restrain it from hurting anyone. It grew from being a cute puppy that drank milk and ate corned beef to a very large German shepherd that ate meat and bones. It was very loyal to us.

I have also in the last decade gone on neighborhood walks with my friend, Peggy who owns a dog called Winnie. The two are always out and about getting their exercise and staying fit. We sometimes drive out for those walks too and feel accomplished when our fitness apps tell us we made 5 kilometers or close to ten thousand steps. Another friend, Susan, and I went on a walk in Bowness Park, Calgary recently. We certainly overdid it; surpassing 6.5 kilometers in just a little over an hour. We had so much to catch up on that we did not realize how far we had walked until our backs began to ache!

I sometimes intersperse my walks with jogging. Somehow my body feels better exercising both upper and lower body in the process and the distance covered is further in a shorter time frame. I set a minimum goal of 2.5 Kilometers and sometimes attach weights to my wrists and or ankles.

It is important to note that one need not run or jog to get fit when dealing with heath challenges like arthritis or heart failure. The most important thing is to keep the body moving however best one can.

SUMMIT AND SADDLE

In general, moderately challenging hiking trails, some of which are trails around Banff National Park and Canmore, are appealing to me. These scenic neighboring towns are just a little over an hour away from me. The area is surrounded by mountains which are spectacular year round, whether it is in the summer or winter months. In Banff for example, my family hiked up the Sulphur Mountain with an elevation of 5,200 feet (1,580 meters) where we took pictures, ate and later got a gondola ride back to ground level. Climbing up that mountain was not an easy feat. Whilst my sons made their way up the mountain with ease, I struggled for breath and was somewhat lightheaded. I stopped intermittently to take slower and deeper breaths and then continued onwards, determined to complete the hike. There are easier hiking trails in the area, for example, the Johnston Canyon Lower Falls section. One doesn't have to engage in difficult trails to attain fitness. Remember, activities need to be fun too.

In 2016, I went on an Israel-Egypt land tour that included a camel-hike up Mount Sinai, Egypt. This hike created some anxiety because it required a reliance on someone else's animal to get me up 7,497 feet (2,285 meters) above sea level. However, the experience itself was great, especially watching the sunrise from the top of the mountain. We also snorkeled in the Red Sea and soaked in the Dead Sea where the mineral is thought to be good for the skin. The snorkeling experience was amazing—the coral was beautiful, and the countless fish in all shapes, color and sizes were breath-taking. I would go back there again, given the chance. The seasoned snorkelers among us believe it has the best sea life and scenery they have ever seen.

We also toured Three Sisters in Blue Mountains, Australia, saw the Wentworth Falls and took lots of pictures. That hike was over 8,000 steps. By the time we returned to Sydney, my watch had recorded well over ten thousand steps that day. I was happy because, even though vacation is usually a time of indulgence for many, I still got my steps in.

Also, the Australian hike around the historic *Three Sisters* and *Wentworth Falls* in the *Blue Mountain* area was very exhilarating. It was truly one of the most amazing hikes ever, with the waterfalls as a bonus; mountains and trees surrounding it.

There are many lovely hiking trails in Alberta where I live and sometimes, I wonder whether the proverb that says *'the grass is always greener on the other side'* holds true in how I'm seeing the world. There is nothing wrong with walking in one's community (except if there are safety concerns) which can be for as long or short as you choose.

GLIDE AND GRACE

When I first visited Canada a week before Christmas 1999, my host and hostess taught me cross country skiing. While it was fun, I fell hard a few times that I began to secretly worry about getting a concussion, despite wearing a helmet the whole time. I also worried about a hip fracture from a fall. I realize that this is one of those excuses that people make when it comes to exercising. We often have a thousand and one reasons why we can't undertake an exercise or activity. This mindset is limiting. If a particular fitness activity doesn't work for you, please consider alternatives from the myriad of options available.

BUILDING YOUR FITNESS HAVEN

Being fit and healthy has been a core value and so exercising regularly is a top priority. The practice of exercise has brought me through stressful periods. Medical research aside, combining brisk walks with jogging provides me with clarity and improved ability to focus. Not exercising for several days leaves me with low energy, body aches from sitting for too long, a feeling that is awful. With exercise, one has a better handle on the stresses of life, including those related to work, like practicing medicine.

The idea of gym membership is often an option for people, and I have tried it too. Gym equipment can appear quite daunting to a novice, so I encourage you to consider getting the guidance of personal trainer for proper exercise routines and appropriate use of equipment to avoid body injury. A trainer can keep one motivated by varying the exercises and introducing one to different equipment each time.

To make gym membership worthwhile and avoid waste of money, I enrolled the whole family at a recreation center near home. This approach increased commitment and accountability. That worked for about three years in the pre-pandemic era when we attended the gym a minimum of twice a week, even on very cold winter days. That practice ended abruptly when the pandemic hit due to the social distancing mandate and the closure of recreational facilities. More recently, the thought of getting dressed for the gym, getting behind wheels to get there has been a deterrent, but has led to a renewed zest for hiking and walks in my neighborhood. There is something about getting outdoors that I find more uplifting than using my home-gym. Though, I prefer the outdoors, the Gym remains an option for me.

It is also important to find out what time of the day works for you to exercise. Being a mom (which means a cook too!) and a full time physician, I find that exercising first thing in the morning works better for me. After work and chores, my energy is too depleted to undergo any exercise later in the day.

Like many others, I feel exercise is important for keeping my weight in check, more so than watching what I eat. Yes, I indulge in the occasional *'sinful foods'*, but that's what they are for me. I drop off the band wagon occasionally and then pick myself back up again.

DANCING LIKE NO ONE'S WATCHING

In the last two years, I've been enjoying dancing as a fitness activity, particularly Zumba. This also means discarding the usual restraint that comes with being an introvert when I attend events where there's music and dancing. The free dance styles that *Afro Beat* music affords me makes it more enjoyable. I made a commitment to myself to always *'dance like no one's watching'* to get a good cardio workout. Dancing gets me in the mood to tackle any problem, literally.

MIND-BODY HARMONY[16,34]

There are many resources online and on bookshelves on the benefits of *Yoga and Pilates*. In the days that I took Pilates and Yoga classes, they were enjoyable. Although some of the poses at the beginner levels appear easy to do, they are great for strengthening and stretching one's muscles. Some of the poses remain part of my exercise routine which combines a few beginner and intermediate poses that improve balance and increase flexibility. For instance, easy poses like the bridge, cat, cobra, and child pose are my favorites for stretching the spine. Single straight leg raises, bicycle and crisscross poses help target the core muscles and back of the legs in the former pose. You might wish to consider **The Pilates Body by Brooke Siler** for more information on how to correctly perform the Pilates poses.[34]

I was bold enough to try hot yoga once, thinking that my tropical origin would help me handle the heat. The yoga studio felt quite hot and it was challenging to keep focused without consistently hydrating myself every so often. Halfway into the yoga poses; one of the attendees threw up and almost passed out. We rallied round her, placed damp towels on her face while she laid on the floor. Although I haven't gone back for hot yoga since them, I believe it could be a great de-stressing physical activity for some.

ENERGY FLOW

I tried the alternative to Chinese Kung Fu, *Qigong*, some years ago which essentially combines physical body movement with controlling one's breath and mental focus (meditation). This was led by a Qigong instructor at a medical women's retreat that took place at Emerald Lake, British Columbia, Canada. The environment itself was serene and the Qigong activity new to me. Although I enjoyed it in the moment, having increased my ability to concentrate and be more mindful, I have not practiced it since then.

The fact that I did not list activities like kick-boxing, barre classes, golfing, swimming, horseback-riding, or whitewater rafting does not mean I do not recommend them. Other than dancing like no one is watching which is similar to Zumba, and the occasional gym time, my all-time favorite fitness activity is hiking combined with a few Pilates and Yoga stretches.

Incorporating fitness into your daily routine not only maintains health, but also helps you reset the stress–burnout button. It is important that you find what types of exercise you find enjoyable and what can be easily incorporated into your unique routine and situations (e.g., health conditions). It needs to be an enjoyable activity for one to be consistent. Not to exercise at all, is a disservice to one's body.

DID YOU KNOW?

Even though aches and pain often follow exercise, they don't last a lifetime. If one gently eases themselves into it, and is consistent, the pain level eventually reduces and can disappear. Walking regularly was helpful when I developed knee pain, and the more consistent, the less the pain level until it disappeared completely. Seriously, it did. I no longer take Acetaminophen or

Ibuprofen on as-needed basis for body aches and pain, it is my cue to resume exercise and be active.

The benefits are simply too many to pass up on. Exercise prevents many diseases, including heart disease, diabetes, hypertension, stroke, cancer, sexual dysfunction, sleep disorder, osteoporosis anxiety, depression, and other mental health conditions. I have benefitted immensely from the practice of using exercise to maintain physical and mental health. I encourage you to give it a short for at least three months to see and reap the benefits.

CULINARY HEALING

Food draws people together and increases the time spent connecting. The trouble is that caution is often thrown to the wind when it comes to ensuring that food ought to be healthy and nutritious. You must agree with me that colorful food that is rich in flavor and lovely to behold is more appealing to the palate than the contrary. Beyond taste and flavor, eating healthy nutritious meals is a strategy for reducing burnout[4].

The relationship between stress and obesity is clear. People often reach for high carbohydrate, high fat foods in times of stress than eat healthy meals or snacks. This is in part due to the hormonal changes that occur from stress, the convenience of these high fat and high carbohydrate foods, or the distraction stress causes and the ensuing mindless eating.

The downside to this is the sluggishness and lack of zeal and energy to exercise or difficulty focusing adequately for long periods of time following the ingestion of high carbohydrates and fats. Moreover, the foods one eats can contribute to ill-health such as hypertension, diabetes, high cholesterol and obesity and its consequences like arthritis in the joints. When one considers the long-term consequences of consuming these high fat and carbohydrate diets, it is imperative to eat healthy foods on a daily basis for the sake of living a good quality life now and in the future.

Find the diet that makes the most sense to you, and avoid fad diets because they are often difficult to adhere to long term.

The *Canada's Food Guide 2019* provides detailed information on why healthy eating is the foundation to health. It states that cardiovascular disease is one of the leading causes of death in Canada. The guide promotes plant-based proteins (e.g. beans, nuts, seeds, tofu, soy) over animal proteins (lean meats, lower fat yogurt), complex carbohydrates (whole grains with high fibre e.g. rice, cereal, bread, pasta), healthier fats (avocado, olive oil, fish) and vegetables and fruits. It also suggests choosing water over other sugary drinks and a reduction in alcohol use.

For teens and adults, the guide recommends an average of 6-8 servings of vegetables and grains, with 2-3 servings of milk and alternative, and meats and alternatives daily. The purpose of the guide is to provide evidence-based advice that helps lower the risks of heart disease, heart attack, hypertension, diabetes, cancers and to promote health.

For more information, please check Canada's food Guide[33] at: *https://food-guide.canada.ca/en/*

The American recommendations are similar to Canadian. In general, the Mediterranean, DASH and Mayo Clinic diet are more flexible than some others and encourage plant-based diet in addition to other food groups, similar to the Canadian food guide. To clarify, the Mayo Clinic diet and Mediterranean diets are diets with healthy lifestyle- focus.[35]

Davis and colleagues share tips on ways one can eat smarter. It notes that to attain optimal health, one needs to avail themselves of over forty nutrients grouped into macronutrients (that is; they form the major bulk of foods comprising carbohydrates, proteins and fats) and micronutrients (minerals and vitamins needed in smaller amounts). MyPyramid (*www.mypyramid.gov*) *is* a United States resource that helps with meal planning that could be useful for maintaining or achieving a healthier weight. There are other resources available to inform the food choices one makes.[29]

I was fortunate in that my mom was an excellent cook, and this spurred my interest in foods and nutrition which was the basis of my ability to maintain my health and weight. She modelled how to cook healthy meals which hopefully have been passed on to the kids. In the process, they may have been spoiled because the food they are used to is colorful, flavorful, and rich in healthy carbohydrates, proteins, and fats, in addition to lots of fruits and veggies. Every other meal follows the same concept.

My uncle recently visited me from the United States and while we were reminiscing about the past, he shared with me how much I loved eating fruits as a little child. He described a kid whose mouth was full and busy biting on a fruit or the other. This was interesting to me because I recall that my mom always bought fruits and ate them daily. If modelling healthy snacking was what she did, then I guess she was successful, since I did develop a love for fresh fruits, and I remember buying them during medical school days from the fruit market by our Anatomy lab.

I understand that others have difficulty accessing and applying nutritional knowledge into every-day life (e.g. financial difficulties), and I feel blessed to have had parents who had the ability to invest in a culture of healthy diet and laid the foundation for my healthy diet and lifestyle. My mother managed a restaurant for the former National Oil Company in the good old days where she made both local and intercontinental dishes. What is your culinary heritage? Are there any old recipes passed down from generations in your family that you would like to teach your children? Now it's your turn.

From my experience as a Family Physician, fruits and vegetables are often lacking in people's diet compared with carbohydrates, protein, and fats, hence, the focus on them in this chapter. When it comes to fruits, I prefer berries, e.g., strawberries, blueberries, blackberries, but not raspberries because of their acidity. One way to avoid the acidity of berries is adding berries to one's yogurt to make a yogurt-fruit parfait. It is important to vary the foods one eats to ensure that one does not lack certain minerals and vitamins; hence, kiwis, pomegranate, grapes, oranges, peaches and plums make the fruit list, especially when in season. Tropical fruits remain my all-time favorites, particularly mangoes, papayas, and pineapple.

What are your favorite fruits? Have you tried stepping out of your comfort zone to try something new and healthy? Do you pay attention to include all food groups in your diet?

I also enjoy eating vegetables like asparagus, the various red, green and orange bell peppers, lettuce, cucumber, peas, carrots, zucchini and squash. I used to think that brussel sprouts were bitter when boiled, until I discovered an alternative way of preparing them. Here is a ***Brussel sprout stir-fry*** recipe you can try:

- *Brussel sprout*
- *Small onion (can be white or red)*
- *A couple of sliced garlic cloves (can skip or use more if desired)*
- *A pinch of salt (add more to taste, depending on the Brussel sprout quantity)*
- *A cup of mixed sliced red and yellow (would skip green bell pepper since Brussel sprout is greenish)*
- *A table spoon of bacon bits (best if lean bacon)*
- *Two table spoons of Olive oil (or alternative)*
- *Sprinkle of black pepper (optional)*

First, wash the Brussel sprout in cold water, trim the stem and remove the outer leaves, then cut up in halves. Thereafter, sauté onion and garlic in olive oil for about five minutes and then add brussel sprouts. Add a sprinkle of salt (black pepper is optional) to taste. Then add the mixed, red bell peppers and bacon bits. If using bacon, remove the excess oil by dabbing it with paper towel.

There are a variety of diet options like *vegetarian diet, vegan diet, Keto Diet, Mediterranean Diet, DASH (Dietary Approaches to Stop Hypertension) diet*, the *MIND diet* which is a combination of Mediterranean and the DASH. More recently there's been some hype regarding intermittent fasting. There are also weight loss programs such as *Weight Watchers* or *Jenny Craig* which seem somewhat more inflexible and appeals to some. My recommendation is balance and portion control, and to avail self of all the food groups, aiming for more fruits and vegetables, nuts (if there are no allergies to them), more whole grains and less saturated fats.

I also can't help but wonder about the role of societal expectation around weight and the stigma associated with being overweight or obese. As a teenager I was self-aware of my appearance. My image problem growing up was being rather skinny, especially after one of my siblings teased that I was *'straight like a stick'*. Since I was in boarding school for High School, I had a pen friend in the United States who was a middle-aged Caucasian woman that I met through a pen pal advertisement in a Christian magazine. I recall asking my pen fried what she thought about a weight gain pill that had been advertised in the same magazine, because I felt there was need to fatten up. She advised against using supplements to increase weight because in her view she felt that with age, the body's metabolism would slow down, and one would wish the opposite at that point. That day did come, and I've become more mindful of what is consumed.

I need to mention the role of festivals and holidays on maintaining a healthy diet. Many times, during celebrations and holidays such as Christmas, Ramadan, Chinese New Year or Hanukkah (and there are many more that have not been listed here), many people throw caution to the wind and indulge in unhealthy food. Across multiple cultures globally, many of these celebrations provide opportunities for social connection, and also feature the addition of more sugary food items on the table; the opposite of what we need to stay healthy. I'm not completely immune from this either. However, if you can select healthier versions of the menu items during your next festive season, your body will thank you.

For Thanksgiving and Christmas, I have a policy of *'strictly Canadian foods on the menu, made from scratch'*. When you cook from scratch, you have the advantage of control over the choice of menu and ingredients so you can regulate the amount of sugar that goes into the desserts and drinks. For Thanksgiving, we typically have two main dishes, rice and a potato dish (e.g. mashed potato or scalloped potatoes), a salad or two, turkey and another protein like fish, appetizers and desserts. For dessert, we usually have traditional pumpkin pie or pecan pumpkin pie. For Christmas, pumpkin pie is swapped for other desserts like fruit cake, pound cake or cheesecake.

We switch things up during Christmas. Eggnog for Christmas dinner was something my kids looked forward to until we began to read food labels more closely. We found out that some eggnog preparations contain some alcohol and were quite high in fat. Though it isn't forbidden, we don't usually buy that anymore, and one can also make eggnog from scratch or purchase healthier versions.

Exercise caution in adopting my personal meal ideas, for I have been told that I have unusual taste buds. For example, I like adding extra nuts, avocado, and berries to everything. Point is, find what you like that is in the same class of food as my examples. Also beware of any dietary restrictions and food intolerances and avoid such.

For breakfast, my go to are:

- *a cup of Greek yogurt topped with blueberries, and or a combination of strawberries, raspberries or blackberries*

- a cup of coffee to which I add a teaspoon or less of honey and
- a dash of cream, or 2 % milk when I'm being more mindful.

Alternatively,

- a slice or two of wholegrain bread with
- a soft-boiled egg (alternative is omelet) and
- a slice of low-fat marbled cheese

Occasionally I would grill these, making a sandwich out of them. And although plain omelet works for me, I enjoy it better when it contains onion, tomato, bell pepper, some spinach, and a pinch of salt to taste.

Lunch is either:

- A mix of berries, with cheese and a handful of nuts, or
- Mixed garden salads as alternatives, to which avocado, strawberries, olives, orange segments, raisins and chicken strips have been added to make it more enjoyable and filling.
- The odd time, a meat pie or sandwich serve as potential lunch substitutes. Processed meat is a no-no, except when very hungry and no alternatives are available to me outside the home.

More often than not, processed meats are avoided due to health concerns around excess salt and gut health. Hence, using real meats like baked chicken for salads or sandwiches are healthier alternatives. These can be made in advance, and stored.

For dinner,

- A protein like chicken, fish or lean red meat, paired with
- A rice dish (rice isn't as boring when one changes it up). Although brown rice is healthier, my preference is Jasmine or Basmati rice, and if I were to cook unflavored rice, a teaspoon of coconut oil or a cup of coconut milk is added to improve the flavor, plus it also has some nutritious better as a healthier alternative to adding butter) and

- *Stir-fry veggies. My favorite vegetables are asparagus, mixed bell peppers, carrots, and peas. Broccoli, cabbage and cauliflower are on the list too, but not as often due to the bloating they cause.*

My version of fried rice requires ingredients like coconut oil instead of canola, or alternatively olive oil; onions and garlic to taste, carrots, green peas, and mushrooms, green, red or orange bell peppers. Sometimes, I sauté shrimps in a tablespoon of heated olive oil and garlic, and later add to the stir-fry. A pinch of rosemary, curry, salt and chicken bouillon (or vegetable-based bouillon, if vegan or vegetarian) to enhance the aroma and flavor. If you are not a fan of rice, quinoa is a healthy substitute.

With the practice of mindful eating, it is easier to maintain consistency in ensuring one's diet is healthy. The more I learn about the benefits of fruits and vegetables over carbohydrates and fats, with some proteins, I feel some guilt eating chocolates or other unhealthy treats.

Some of the harms of high calorie foods and simple sugars have been mentioned in the earlier part of the discourse e.g., dental caries, heart disease, and wide sugar swings that increase the chance of irritability for those with attention deficit and hyperactivity disorder (**ADHD**). The key message is that one needs to remember that eating well today contributes to a better health tomorrow.

Here is my invitation to please come on board and let's join forces to keep each other accountable.

BONUS

Other than health benefits, healthy diet consisting of vegetables and fruits are high in oxidants and are essential for good skin and anti-aging. The trick is the more colorful and varied these food items are, the better for one's health. Occasionally, compliments are sent my way regarding my youthfulness. This is one of my secrets, outside of genetics and physical fitness.

HYDRATE TO HEAL[32,33]

Water is best over other beverages. Historically, the average water intake stipulated has been *six to eight* glasses per day to maintain hydration. This might not be feasible for those with certain health conditions for instance, heart or kidney failure or in the elderly where there's been an altered sense of thirst coupled with urinary incontinence. The Canada Food guide recommends water over sugary beverages.[33]

The recommendation for alcohol consumption is two drinks for males and one drink for females, but it's beneficial if you consume zero alcohol most days. I recommend abstaining from alcohol due to the new discoveries of its link with certain types of cancer. A middle ground could be weekly alcoholic beverage, bearing in mind that limiting alcoholic beverages is not a challenge for me as it might be for others, thanks to mom who could not handle alcohol, unless it was a mild aperitif such as *St. Raphael's* or *Dubonnet Tonic Wine*. Anything stronger in terms of alcoholic content she avoided like a plague. She mentioned that she felt the alcohol hit her brain with the very first sip. I happen to be that way too; needing to dilute wine with *Ginger Ale* and rarely able to consume a full 6 oz. wine serving. It's okay if you call my drink sangria because of the dilution.

BUZZ AND BURNOUT

Caffeine has some health benefits, including being high in antioxidants which prevent certain types of cancers. It can also be used to stay alert, potentially reducing work errors or motor vehicle accidents. However, it also has the potential to cause certain health problems when ingested in excess, because it is a stimulant. Ideally, the daily caffeine intake should be limited to 2-3 cups, as higher amounts have been linked with osteoporosis (thinning of the bone), high blood pressure), and disruptive sleep when consumed close to bedtime.

Tips:

- *May consume 1-3 cups of coffee/day for some health benefits, if there are no contraindications*
- *Avoid drinking coffee late in the afternoon to prevent sleep disruption*

SUBSTANCES[32]

Many people use recreational substances to increase energy levels, manage sleep disturbances or boost confidence level. However, the harms associated with these substances are much higher than any temporary benefit of feeling relaxed, ability to overcome anxiety in social settings, or fall asleep faster. I grew up in a home where there was no tobacco or other substances, except alcohol on social basis when my dad's friends were visiting him at the house. As far as recalled, there was no excessive use of alcohol. One day however, I got back from school in Grade 6 (elementary school) and saw my dad smoking cigarettes. After greeting him and walking away, my inquisitive mind would not let me be until I got out pen and paper and began to write down the thoughts that came. In my three-page write-up, addressed to dad, I expressed my disappointment.

I worried about how dad would perceive this letter, so I handed it over to one of dad's co-workers who was meeting up with him later that day before a trip. I was at unrest until he returned. As soon as I heard his voice, I went into hiding, much like the Adam and Eve story recounted in the Bible. I could not hide for long because he had a tradition of calling out *'all my children line up!'* each time he returned from a trip. So, I cowered out of my hiding place. To this day, I am glad he did not keep me in suspense about what his thoughts were, because I had suffered terribly thinking the worst. I mean, I was not the only child of his who had seen him smoking cigarettes that day. To make matters worse, I acted in isolation and had not sought the input of my siblings before sending off the letter. This was a solo health match in a battle with an adult; my father; whose choice I had questioned.

Long story short, dad started the family meeting by announcing that he received the letter I had written him about not smoking cigarettes. He shared that when my letter arrived his table, he was smoking another cigarette from his brand-new Benson and Hedges package which he seemed to be enjoying. According to him, the last puff he had taken before reading my letter was his very last. He discarded the rest of the package. Although he was feared for his mostly authoritarian stance, he apologized to us and never smoked again until his death many decades later.

Some use substances from peer pressure, or to simply have fun. However, I think that with substances, the harm outweighs the benefits. You should have fun without harming your body.

I also do not recommend use of marijuana, except it is medically necessary, such as when conventional treatment fail, or part of palliative care. I have always held a strong view against the use of addictive substances as early on in life as I remember. My view should not be your principle. Please do a comprehensive benefits-risk review of any substance you desire to use.

MAINTAINING PEAK PHYSICAL HEALTH[36]

Ensuring that one has a trusted primary care provider, example, a Family Physician, is essential to healthy living, aside from nutritious diet, exercise and mental health tune ups. The practice of preventative health is vital to living well, and the sooner one starts making those changes, the more the benefits.

Please start today, and not later than tomorrow to book a well-check appointment.

Despite the divide around the recommended timing and the usefulness of cancer screening, I'm an advocate for preventative health measures. For example, in Alberta, Canada, the earliest age for cervical cancer screening is age 25; with the consideration to start three years after being sexually active for the female who is yet to be sexually active by age 25. Breast cancer screening guideline is now being offered earlier as the benefit of early detection outweighs the risks associated with radiation exposure. Current guidelines says to start at age 45. However, with a positive family history of breast cancer in first degree relatives, it is recommended to start even earlier.

The discomfort associated with the mammogram is often cited as a reason to skip this test. I agree that it is rather uncomfortable. Balancing the discomfort associated with mammogram, with the benefit of early diagnosis and treatment to avert severe consequences (such as cancer-related death), makes it a worthwhile venture in my view. For those identifying as women, there are other reproductive cancers like cervical cancer, ovarian cancer or uterine cancer, or prostate cancer or testicular cancer for those who have those organs. Breast cancer screening mainly targets females, but men with family history of male breast cancer may want to consider having the screening conversation with their family doctors.

By the age of fifty, individuals are encouraged to screen for colon cancer too. A former university graduate of mine lost his life to colon cancer a few years before turning fifty. When in doubt or for unexplainable persistent bowel changes, please book an appointment with your primary care provider.

Also, low dose lung CT scan is now being offered to those with a history of chronic tobacco use who may be at a higher risk for lung cancer.

For general advice on when and where to go for screening, please check *Screening for life* website: *https://screeningforlife.ca/* Please check your jurisdiction for resources and guides that apply to you.

Other than cancer screening there are other diseases that need to be tested that are quite important for individuals to adhere to. This includes high blood pressure checks, diabetes screening, cholesterol screening, thyroid dysfunction especially with symptoms suggestive of change, and osteoporosis screening as people get older. The family physician is there as a guide for when these tests are appropriate.

GENETICS AND MEDICATION COMPLIANCE

This chapter would be incomplete without sharing the need to consider being medication-compliant when diagnosed with treatable health conditions. As is evident, not everyone with hypertension or diabetes was negligent about their diet or fitness. For example, my mom believed she did not need to take pills because of her spiritual beliefs; hoping for the miracle of healing. Many people like my mom do not trust orthodox medicine, some based out of fear and worry about side effects, and others due to mistrust of the pharmaceutical companies and doctors in general.

I remember a time my mom came to visit me at the university and during our conversation shared that she had been having headaches quite consistently. We presented at an outpatient clinic where her blood pressure was checked and it read *220/120 mmHg* repeatedly. She was prescribed anti-hypertensive medication which she refused to take on faith grounds. She desperately wished to be healed through prayer and was non-compliant with her prescribed anti-hypertensive medications, until she suffered a stroke; a complication of uncontrolled high blood pressure. Sadly, the by the time she agreed to take her medications regularly, the harm had already been done.

High blood pressure can kill, and so can many untreated diseases. In the case of high blood pressure or diabetes, when they do not kill out rightly, they put strain on organs like the heart, kidneys and the brain and nerves. Unfortunately, once these organs are damaged, treatment only aims to preserve their current function as reversal is no longer possible.

Although genetics has a role in one's health, a routine that is consistent in ensuring fitness, healthy diet, adequate water intake (about 6-8 glasses a day), limited alcohol consumption (four or less alcoholic beverages per week regardless of gender), adequate sleep (7-9 hours/day) go a long way in keeping individuals not just fit and healthy, but also younger, happier with the potential for a disease-free aging. Be mindful about the benefits of exercise and healthy food. This goes a long way in maintaining a consistent routine for overall wellness and health maintenance.

It is often said *'you are what you eat'* which some say is a derogatory clause, even though it might be somewhat true. Hence, *'I will eat healthy because my body deserves to be nourished with the right foods and drinks for a healthier me and better aging.'*

Join me.

REFLECTION QUESTIONS

Do you make time for exercise? How often in a week do you exercise? What kind of exercise do you engage in? Do you incorporate weights (strengthening) and cardiovascular or aerobics into your fitness routine? Do you have a gym membership? How committed are you with attendance? What needs to change to allow you commit to regular usage? Have you considered the use of a fitness instructor?

FITNESS

1. Write the benefits of exercise down.
2. Is fitness one of your values? If so, what do you do to maintain your fitness?
3. If not, how might you enjoy moving your body with the intention of improved mental wellbeing? What is standing in your way?
4. Are you willing and able to make a commitment to yourself to invest in your physical health?
5. If you plan to start now, write what you plan to do, how often and the specific time of the day.
6. How will you measure success?

FOOD

Do you eat balanced healthy and nutritious meals each day? Does this include greens, yellow and orange vegetables? How about fruits? How about meats and plant proteins, carbohydrates (carbs) and fats? What stops you from eating a wholesome and nutritious meal? What can you do to change that?

1. What is your attitude towards food? Do you believe that food should be enjoyable, even if it means they are unhealthy?
2. Would you make room for dessert whenever you eat out ? Or would you remind yourself that you are full and

do not have to make room for dessert? Could you, for instance, take the dessert home rather than eat it even when there is no room in one's belly?
3. What would it take to change your relationship with food and beverages you ingest?

WEIGHT AND HEALTH

What is your ideal body weight? How did you arrive at that weight ideal? Have you discussed your ideal with a professional or done the research on the topic? What would it take to get closer to your ideal body? Are you abstaining from certain foods, practicing intermittent fasting or engaging in other fad diets? How successful has it been for you? If anything but successful, who have you turned to for professional help e.g., dietitian, fitness coach, family physician, or physiotherapist?

SLEEP

Do you have a set time for sleep each night? Is this consistent or inconsistent? Do you have a pre-sleep routine? What does it consist of? How is that going for you? Is there anything you need to change to achieve more consistency? How many hours do you sleep at night? Do you experience sleep disruptions? What is contributing to disrupted sleep, if any e.g. room temperature, room environment with distractors, bed or bedding, pillows, or partner issues like snoring?

Do you wake up feeling refreshed in the morning? What might be interfering with your sleep? Do you have symptoms of pain in the joints or muscles, headaches, frequent urination, hot flushes, restless legs, muscle cramps to name a few? Has anyone told you that you snore? Have you checked this out with your family doctor or sleep physician? Have you been diagnosed with sleep apnea? What have you done about it? Do you have the equipment and not use it? What is posing a barrier to your regular usage e.g., appliance type, fitting issues? What are the advantages and disadvantages of using a seep machine? What would it take to commit to improving your sleep and your overall health?

Addendum

1. Assuming the answers to the above questions show these are not an issue for you, what is keeping you awake?
2. Are you worried about things or work or family?
3. Would you say you are a worrier? How would others in your social circle describe you?

Tip: Perhaps consider scheduling an appointment with a healthcare professional about possible mood issues like anxiety or depression, or other medical conditions that could disrupt sleep at night?

CHAPTER SEVEN

THE POWER OF SOCIAL CONNECTIONS

HEALING THROUGH COMMUNITY[4,27,37,38]

It is often said that humans are social beings and are hard-wired to connect and interact with others. To not do so, is a recipe for disaster. There are several opportunities for individuals to connect with others; starting from the home front to workplaces, and the wider community. In professions like medicine, peer supports have been effective in reducing the social isolation that can often result. The type of connections formed vary from the more informal to formal through Balint groups, Practice-Based Small Groups, and other Continuing Medical Education opportunities.[37,38] Some physicians tackle the challenges of medical practice using Narrative and Appreciative Inquiry Exercises, which fosters interpersonal self-awareness; comprising the awareness of relationships and communication. Each weekly session starts with a theme that participants focus on while writing brief stories about their personal experiences in medical practice, combined with appreciative inquiry techniques to explore ways they successfully managed difficult clinical situations. They also highlight the personal qualities that brought about the success. The goal of focusing on the reinforcement of positive experiences changes behavior in desired directions than exploring negative experiences or gaps.[16]

In this chapter, I discuss some of my attempts at building my own community from elementary and later in life.

BUILDING MY FIRST COMMUNITY

In grade 5, I formed a club in elementary school called the *'Intelligent Girls Club' (IGC)*. This club had approximately fifteen members. I thought it was a neat idea to form a group of like-minded individuals who were goal oriented. It seemed we all had a similar passion to excel at the time. Everyone I had approached to join the club obliged after presenting a case for a group of people with similar interests and indomitable presence. I guess I learned early in life that *'we are stronger together'*. I really couldn't say, but there is a chance that this was also one way to handle the bullying I had experienced in Grade 2 to 3, a situation that seemed to have lasted a lifetime, until I mustered courage to inform my class teacher.

I was the president of the club, and we had roles and responsibilities defined for vice president, treasurer and secretary as well. There was a weekly schedule which was rotated to keep things interesting. The games we played were well-planned. At the end of elementary school, we organized our own group photos and paid the school photographer out of pocket. We went our different ways thereafter.

THE PHYSICIAN SISTERS COMMUNITY, CALGARY

In the last seven years, I have grown a small community of female physician friends with similar interests. We hang out together, dine together, attend and support one another at community events, laugh and share stories about our personal and professional experiences. We celebrate life and support one another through difficulty, such as the death of a loved one in a group member's family. We ensure there are no unrealistic expectations held; rather focusing on being our authentic selves, demonstrating mutual respect and freedom of speech and ideas. This is similar to what is described as *'Commensality Groups'* which is a burnout mitigation strategy for physicians supported by some studies.

Outside of the physician group, there are a few non- physician friends that I spend time with; some are walking buddies, movie buddies, and with one or more attend concerts, or museum shows like van Gogh show in Calgary, 2022. With one or more we share celebrations like thanksgiving and Christmas dinners. I consider myself blessed to have trusted friends and colleagues to do life with together. That network has grown and continues to grow. This also doesn't suggest that all friendships are rosy. The ones that stand the test of time are the best.

Within my family, I have a few confidants as well, connecting as often as possible, given time zone differences. These are people with whom I am vulnerable because they care genuinely. Despite their inability to help me navigate certain challenges being several thousands of miles apart, they remain a wellbeing buffer. Don't get me wrong, we also have our fair share of family drama, given the different personalities and perspectives.

Around the 2020 COVID-pandemic, I re-established contact with my paternal second cousin who resides in the U.S.A. I call him *uncle* because of the age gap between us; at almost two decades. We chat about just about anything. He is always advising, sharing words of wisdom and encouragement. I also learned that he had been very close with my mom who has since passed away. He had donated a pint of his blood when my mom experienced post-partum hemorrhage, following the birth of my younger brother; the fifth of my mom's children.

The fact that he considered donating blood back in the early 1970s means a lot to me; that he cared enough about family; and mom. This suggested that there was a sense of community within our family. The Igbo culture of my dad's people is such that if one marries a wife, she becomes everybody's wife; as in those within the family. It means she treats them well and they do the same as they would their own wives.

There are also a couple of cousins who grew up with me in dad's house with whom I have maintained some contact. Social media platforms like Facebook, Instagram and WhatsApp have helped a lot in making that possible. Up until a couple of decades ago, we wrote letters and depended on the postal service to deliver mails. Oftentimes the postal service was unreliable; if not outright impossible to deliver mail because many houses in various Nigerian cities do not have assigned postal codes.

That said, social media has erased the need for long wait times for mail delivery. Messages get delivered instantly, and with social media apps and cell phone internet service, one can make calls without extra charges almost worldwide.

PRACTICE BASED SMALL GROUP

In terms of professional network, I also joined a Practice Based Small group with a few colleagues who are Family Physicians. We meet monthly to share professional experiences, review a module of interest and attempt to answer the assigned case-based questions. Other than networking, we claim continuing medical education credits for the modules upon completion. The timing of the meeting isn't always conducive but remains valuable. Ours is through McMaster University, which is one of many programs offering the service.

As the saying goes, *'no man is an island'*. The social network helps keep me in balance.

CONNECT WITH YOUNGER SELF

This section is about all the little things we did when we were younger, curious, more daring sometimes and hopefully happier. Can you think about those times when as kids one goofed around and didn't take life so seriously? When our friends could offend us and we forgave them instantly. It is those activities that can pull us out of our shells into that happy place, if we would create time for them. It is important to note however, that some childhood memories are not without trauma, so please reflect upon those, only if it feels safe for you to.

It is important to address traumatic childhood and adulthood experiences, and attend to our emotional health if they have been unattended to until this point in time. The importance of this is that the brain does need to heal for us to function and relate with others better. This will be discussed further under the need for professional care (therapy).

CREATIVE THERAPIES

As a kid, we often visited zoos, ate out, watched movies on T.V or in the movie theatres and visited with friends and family. Although watching movies on a regular basis is impossible, due to there being 'no time', it is a relaxing activity. So, when I travelled to Australia this last summer, a trip that was almost fifteen hours long, airport-to-airport, much of the flight time was spent sleeping and listening to music. The trip allowed me some space to connect with my younger self, with no care in the world. This absence of care in the world was possible because my colleagues had agreed to provide coverage in my absence. Although there were some hiccups during the first two days of travel, those were soon replaced with excitement about learning about other people and their ways of life.

During the plane ride, I journaled and watched three movies, one of which was Magic Mike's last dance which was quite a movie, with sensual dancing and the finding of self and love between the two main characters; Maxmara and Mike. They had agreed to work together to spice up what appeared to be a rather dull drama act that Max's ex- husband's family had been running for decades out of a theatre the family owned. Mike was a lap dancer who was lured into doing a last dance by Max who had promised to pay him $60,000 to direct the drama at their theatre. Although there were hiccups along the way, I thought it was well done.

The other movie *'Wanna Dance'* was about the late Whitney Houston. Whitney died at an early, which the media says was substance-related. She had been one of my music icons and it was interesting to watch a biopic of her life. She was certainly a legend, and her death a loss to the world of a great legend. The first Black American to win seven Grammy awards, she outpaced The Beatles, and the late Michael Jackson who himself was a Black American who achieved stardom at a tender age.

Whitney's death reminds one of how so ephemeral life can be. I remember to be grateful that despite the many challenges one has faced, being alive and well and financially stable is a gift.

In Sydney, Australia, I visited the Bondi Beach, Sydney Olympic Park, restaurants, and did some shopping. Cairns, Australia was also great to visit, even though it just about rained the whole time reminding me of the United Kingdom. I enjoyed visiting Palm Cove beach and sampled wares from the local market. Not sure why, I also bought a red wrap for belly dancing. To think I'd visited Dubai twice and never bought this item is a marvel. Reflecting further, I see a connection to my childhood when we would sometimes find a wrapper to tie around our waist and dance to the local music. We will see how I make out trying belly dancing which is one of the things on my to-do list within the year. Through this, I felt as though I connected with my younger self who was often mischievous back in the day.

The boat trip to the Great Barrier Reef, Cairns was not smooth at all. Almost half the passengers were seasick with the turbulent waves encountered. The boat staff appeared unperturbed as they efficiently distributed bags to passengers who needed to throw up. No one from my party vomited, although some of us felt slightly nauseous. Our secret was that we had all taken *Gravol* (Metoclopramide) tablets before the boat took off.

The Reef itself was wonderful with underwater sights consisting of fish and sea plants. I attempted snorkeling but did not last long in the water. My guide was *'baby Alicia'* who is now in her early twenties. I just couldn't see her as my guide even though she had taken her mom with her before me. There were other reasons I didn't participate. Perhaps, I was distracted because the original plan was to host an *Instagram* event while on the sea. This didn't happen due to unstable internet. Lunch on the boat was excellent, with a variety of tasty food items.

Our last day in Australia was spent at the Sydney Zoo where just about all animals are housed. There was a wide range of animals from Africa, Asia and Australia. There were a variety of snakes, including green python, and other animals and birds like kangaroo, emu, giraffe, cheetah, tiger, lion, elephants, crocodile, and koalas. The habitats of these animals have been replicated quite successfully. The koala for one was found sleeping on a Eucalyptus tree in which it feeds. Pretty much all the koalas were found doing what they knew best, eating and sleeping for long hours. The thought is they are dormant because they do not get enough nutrition from eating eucalyptus leaves. They then sleep for long hours to conserve their energy.

Since the next day was the return trip to Canada, I stayed with my host, at a hotel close by the airport to avoid any morning traffic congestion. My friend like me, is always on the go, perhaps more than I've been able to. She seems to have vacations all planned out well in advance and as often as is feasible, considering the kids' school calendars.

There are other activities one could do that could help individuals connect with their younger self. For instance, I was at a friend's cabin in 2022 and she had rock painting supplies. By the time we realized it, we had spent over two hours painting until past ten at night. I had wholly immersed myself into the activity, and so did my daughter. While I painted a butterfly on a rock, she painted beach-side scenery.

Connect with your younger self, no matter what it takes. It is an opportunity to rejuvenate and recharge. It allows the beauty and youth inside you to float to the surface. Connecting with your younger self means being daring, letting go, leading with curiosity and enjoying life to the fullest in the moment.

I also reconnected with my younger self, when I went biking with a friend in the neighborhood. That exercise took me back to my childhood days, and it was exhilarating.

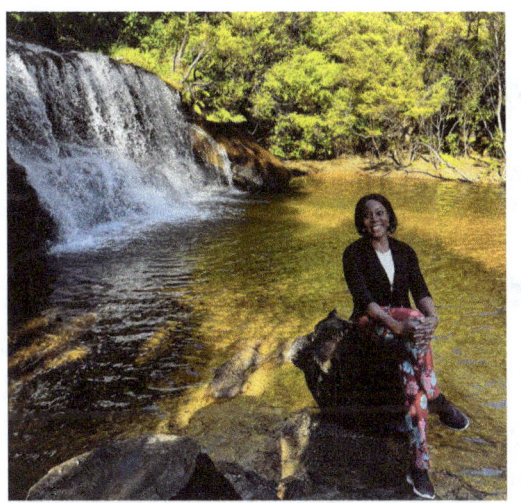
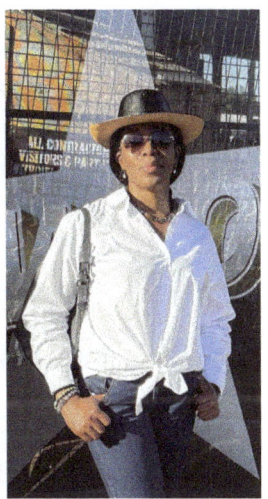
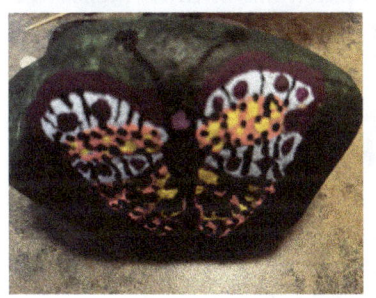
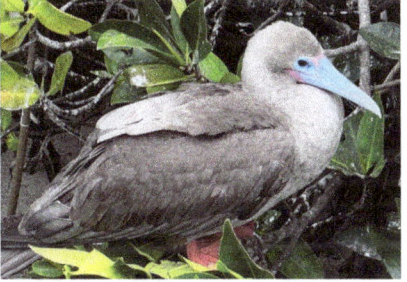

Top Left: Visitng Wentworth Falls, Blue Mountains, Australia. Top Right: Stepping out of my comfort zone, to attend the World Famous Calgary Stampede in 2022. Bottom - Left: Rock Painting of a butterfly. Bottom-Right: Visiting Blue Boobies in Galapagos, Ecuador

REFLECTION QUESTIONS

CONNECTING WITH YOUR YOUNGER SELF

1. Do you recall who your younger self was?
2. Did you like your younger self? If you did, what will it take for you to connect with your younger self again?
3. If you did not have great experiences as a younger person, what would you have wanted your younger self to have had? What would it take to make that happen?

SOCIAL CONNECTIONS

1. What was growing up like for you?
2. Who do you consider to be in your inner circle of friends or confidantes?
3. What is standing in your way of expanding your social circle? What are the potential benefits or drawbacks from trusting and being open to new social connections?

CHAPTER EIGHT

THE GIFT OF SPIRITUALITY

TAPPING INTO HIGHER POWERS[4]

Ann Masten explained resilience as *reflecting the resources and processes that individuals applied to restore equilibrium, counter challenges, or transform themselves.*[39] This means that your choice of resources and processes will vary from mine and the next person.

The key is choosing wisely from the different enriching resources available to you. For me it is the *physical, the mental and the spiritual.*[23]

This section is not an attempt to endorse one belief over another. It also does not imply throwing caution to the wind, as not every spiritual leader practices what is being preached. Seek the truth about spirituality and see if it's a strategy you might consider at some point, almost the same way one considers a counsellor. For instance, my personal experience with spiritual leaders has not always been positive. Somehow, I've managed to move myself from the point of dependency on any one spiritual leader to focusing on my relationship with the Creator. I am also able to study the Bible myself and apply it as best as I can to my day-to-day living.

This chapter aims to place value on the power of spirituality in getting people through challenging times. It does not mean that everything will be perfect because one is spiritually inclined; rather it means that even amid challenges one takes solace knowing that the phase will yet pass. People who have faith in the supernatural are often better able to move from the place of despair to one of acceptance and ultimately reliance.

A preacher shared that without a sense of hope and joy, despair can drive people to death by suicide because they cease to see a reason for living. The suggestion was for individuals to anchor themselves in a passage of their spiritual book; example the Bible or other such books. That preacher finds that he gets solace and encouragement when faced with difficulties reading the Bible passage in 1st John 5: 4 which states: *'for everyone born of God overcomes the world. This is the victory that has overcome the world, even our faith'*.

He also shared something I felt was interesting. He believes that one need not be a Christian to progress in life; that is, provided one is investing time and energy for the general good of others, they will advance.

From my personal experience, if it wasn't for the Creator; I wouldn't be a Physician and would not be here today to share my stories or ideas. Here is how I came to this conclusion:

The country of my birth is such a beautiful place with wonderful people, and at the same time, unfortunately, there are some bad eggs there too. I experienced a near-kidnap situation in my fifth year of medical school that no one could have imagined. It began as an innocent conversation with a lady I encountered on my way back to my residence which was off campus. She invited me to try for modelling for a product she claimed she was marketing. I did not realize that I was walking into the lion's den.

Upon entry of this uncompleted building, I realized my folly. Long story short, it took silently praying throughout my interaction with these two men and unknown woman for me to leave that den. They kept me there for several hours until it was nightfall asking me to provide them with gold, cash and anything else that they felt I might have. Intermittently the leader would ask me why I appeared calm, after they had tried several ways of extracting money from me. They first showed me how they were able to print cash and how I could be very rich overnight. It required I would contribute some money in getting the chemicals needed.

I told them that I was content with what I had and was uncomfortable with the idea. At the end of it all, I was let go. There were no neighbors, nothing. It was a building in an isolated place. And I just happened to be fasting that day. In my mind this was not supposed to happen on a day like this. But then, I think the key learning is that I was protected from these three individuals and for that, I lean into the Creator even more.

The point of this chapter is to encourage you to draw on your spirituality regularly. While praying, ensure you are present. This does not mean that you longer have one or two distracting thoughts, but you have the ability to catch yourself and re-center your mind.

My relationship with the Creator centers me because it is one of my strongest values. It helps me put others first. In fact, in serving others, I gain strength to do what I could not ordinarily do for myself. A relationship with God does not prevent you from facing life's challenges. However, when those challenges come, you will be able to draw strength that will help you weather the storms. A friend of mine once said, *"life does not privy us to control* it, rather roll with it; the biggest factor of longevity is who with, and how we travel it."

I also remind myself of Bible passages that speak to calmness and peace such as *'Be still and know I am God...'* (Psalm 46:10) — this is a meditative passage that helps ground me. The passage says to be still, regardless of what life throws at me. The other aspect of the passage says *'and know that I am God.'* By reminding myself that I have a spiritual Father who cares about me, I'm better able to let go of hurts. I also take solace in knowing that sometimes negative things occur to the best of us, but in those times, I have learned not to question but to reflect and ponder, seeking what learning there is from it all. In the end, I pray and leave it with the Creator.

The Bible passage Romans 8:20 that says *'everything is working out for the good of those who love God;'* is one that I sometimes find difficult to accept depending on the situation. This is partly because it is anything but good when one loses their job, a family member or friend, especially if unexpected. But in the faith journey, we can question but we don't always have an answer. The key point about being spiritually inclined is that one is more likely to accept what one can't control or change, leaving it with the higher powers to address one way or the other. However, I have seen or heard stories of people who were laid off work only to land better jobs.

A day before writing this chapter, I had a near-miss with death from what would have been considered a fatal accident. I had been invited to give a mental health talk in downtown Calgary that day. I got to the area about thirty minutes before the start of the event. It was while looking for the building's underground parking without success that I resorted to calling the coordinator of the event who began to give me directions. That direction led me on to a train track! No sooner had I ventured onto the track did I notice a train coming right behind me.

In a split second I pulled over into a rather high concrete pavement with two trees planted barely a couple of feet away, just enough space for my vehicle to maneuver in between. It also began to rain dogs and cats at the same time. After what seemed like eternity, a security guard tried to help by looking out to see if there were any other trains coming. When it was safe to get off the pavement on to the track again, I did a quick u-turn to leave the area. There was no time to process the event after narrowly escaping a train-car accident, I was glad and full of gratitude for the privilege to be alive and deliver the mental health workshop tasked with.

In fact, that experience made me reflect on how ephemeral life can be. *Here today, gone tomorrow* as they say. Gone like a wind, or a withered grass. I had also just learned about an alumnus of ours from medical school who passed away on the weekend. I was older than him by a good five years! Looking at his pictures, he was full of life, still relatively young and promising. He left behind a wife and two young kids. How saddening. I mean it could have been me, were that train going at a much faster speed. My conclusion was that someone must have been watching out for me. Now, I'm mindful of that view because it doesn't mean those who passed away from accidents or other health conditions did not have someone watching over them.

Beyond my own personal experiences as it relates to spirituality, there are a couple of pastors that I connect with on a spiritual level. During my writing, one of them shared some strategies employed for mitigating burnout and self-accountability as a spiritual leader. Examples are scheduling retreat time quarterly, having a day of rest for self-care (synonymous with mental health day) where no other work is done, spending time in meditation and listening to other inspiring spiritual leaders to equip self, and making time for family as well. I was curious about how spiritual leaders take care of themselves to prevent burnout, because as one can imagine, they too are caregivers to their members.

They are the ones people turn to when things go wrong in their private lives and are likely to learn of people's personal challenges on a larger scale and deeper level than the average person (aside from physicians or counsellors).

Another pastor I happen to connect with quite often acknowledged their frailty and humanity during our one –on-one. The individual's practice is to start each encounter with gratitude for the gift of life and other blessings. For instance, one could express gratitude for the gift of family, friends, ability to provide for one's family the basic needs of life (food, clothing, and shelter), good health and other achievements and successes. If need be, this may be followed by prayers for a specific need to be met or clarity and guidance while embarking on projects or other endeavors.

In terms of dealing with workplace stresses or burnout, spirituality has benefits for the the individual who identifies it as their core value. The practice of meditative prayer allows the individual to channel positive energy in all they do, work on reducing negativity, and hopefully be able to overcome obstacles in their way. This does not mean that those who are not spiritually inclined are not able to overcome adversity or other struggles. It also doesn't mean that those who are spiritually inclined are free from those curveballs life throws at us.

The short form of **Serendipity Prayer** written by the American Theologian, Reinhold Niebuhr in the 1930s could serve as a useful meditative piece for dealing with anxiety or other stressful situations:

> *"Lord, grant me the strength to accept the things I cannot change, the courage to change the things I can, and the wisdom to know the difference."*
> — *Dr. Reinhold Niebuhr*

REFLECTION QUESTIONS

1. What does spirituality mean to you?
2. Do you see any benefits to applying spiritual lens to life?
3. Have you had negative experiences with spiritual leaders? How have you dealt with that?
4. Do you think it might be worth it to trust again- example, the Creator, spiritual leaders? Why, or why not?

Tip:

- *Engaging in the spiritual practice of renewal does not equate with religiosity. One can be spiritually inclined without associating with any one religious sect.*
- *Meditative mindfulness expressed as spirituality isn't about the benefits that accrue one, rather an honest desire for an intimate relationship with one's creator and the willingness to practice self-lessness.*
- *For those who practice intermittent fasting for weight management, how about considering meditative mindfulness to get the most benefit physically, mentally, spiritually and possibly socially.*

CHAPTER NINE

THE COURAGE TO DO IT DIFFERENTLY

RECOVER & REBUILD WITH PROFESSIONAL CARE

Burnout and its root causes and the consequences have been identified through various lenses; personal experiences, clients' stories and the literature. Recovery from burnout will also take different approaches for different individuals because we are all unique in our own ways.

This chapter aims to discuss some aspects around professional care. Professional care on its own would be insufficient without incorporating personal and workplace elements. Hence, managers and other leaders, and human resources personnel need to liaise together to ensure that the worker experiencing burnout can return to a better work environment and thrive. Strategies that managers or leaders can take have already been addressed in chapter four.

THE ROLE OF PRIMARY CARE PROVIDERS AND THERAPISTS

While it is great to surround one with trusted family members and friends, a majority are not in the position to assist others heal adequately from burnout. This is true in part from not being trained in this area of work and the fact that the existing ties could blur the boundary lines and inadvertently create other issues. This comment isn't meant to solicit for clients needing therapy rather, demonstrate the objective truth about the time, energy and ability to apply a *trauma-informed* approach to therapy. I would suggest that a trip to one's primary care provider; be it a family physician or nurse practitioner could be a good starting point.

Burnout is not the only reason for energy depletion and emotional exhaustion. There is a myriad of physical and mental health conditions that mimic burnout. For example: anxiety, depression, thyroid disorders, Vitamin B12 deficiency, chronic fatigue syndrome, sleep apnea, undiagnosed cancer, or undiagnosed Diabetes. Work with your primary care provider to rule out other causes of severe fatigue, especially if your symptoms do not go away in a short time interval (two to four weeks.) I advise making an appointment with your primary care provider early. However, the next best time is now. Better late than never.

Recovery requires a multi-pronged approach, besides strategies that the individual can incorporate such as lifestyle changes which are often insufficient in addressing burnout fully. Although burnout is not a mental health disorder, psychological therapists have a role to play aside from physicians and nurse practitioners. Therapists are trained psychologists who are able to assist people with their journey through wellness in general. The role of a therapist in burnout journey is to holistically review both the work and personal aspects of the individual's life to target the ills of culture where they exist as well as the role of personal habits and lifestyles. To be comprehensive also requires healthy workplace practices, in addition to boundary-setting, acknowledging and gradually challenging all forms of distorted cognitive thinking and intentionally incorporating mindfulness, and the practice of self-compassion and gratitude into one's daily routines.

Sometimes there is a need to tackle certain issues from scratch, and other times a modification suffices. For instance, in Carla's case, it was important that to reset she needed to take time off work. Carla had struggled with guilt regarding being off work, asking, *'but who will do the job, and how will my co-workers cope if I don't show up to work?'* She was more worried about the organization's ability to cope given the healthcare worker shortages experienced locally and globally. She was advised to have that conversation with her family doctor. She did.

While off work, she was encouraged to work on improving her sleep hygiene, continue eating a healthy diet and exercising regularly, which were some examples of things she could do within her locus of control. My psychologist friend, Susan Hastie, says *'socializing happens when our nervous system is healthy and free from competing stressors, where the self is not contained and marginalized by the constraints brought on by stress such that the posture movement required to socialize is unavailable.'*

She also began to create time to network with her social contacts in the community, something she was unable to bring herself to do due to the sheer exhaustion she had experienced for many consecutive months prior. She had shared that while burned out, she was more cynical, self-loathing and began self-isolating, and had canceled many social function opportunities because she had no energy reserve to draw from. She did not see the sense in even bothering anymore. Carla was not a weak person; she was the epitome of resilience. She drew some strength from the spiritual connection felt whenever she was out and about in nature.

Carla also had a discussion with her manager regarding her work schedule as a driver negatively impacting her physical and mental wellbeing. Together with her manager, they set clearer definition of her roles and responsibilities. On occasion however, she continues to provide coverage whenever they were short of staff. She had also made some hard decisions regarding her ability to thrive in the organization in the event the organization could not accommodate her wellness needs. Examples include less frequent unilateral work schedule changes, having a day a week where she could attend to her physical health needs since her schedule is such that her hours strapped morning and evening hours, and a weekend day.

Unfortunately, Kai on the other hand was let go by his organization partly due to organizational restructuring and the irritability as behavioral consequence of burnout. Kai began his healing with his family doctor and later tagged on the therapy. He went through two psychological therapists before he felt he was beginning to heal and recover. It is not unusual to have to try out mental health therapists before settling with one with whom one feels a connection. The same is true of any primary care provider or other professionals.

Although Kai reflected on the burnout repercussions on his behavior and felt some guilt, he was able to practice forgiveness for those who caused him some emotional injury at work, and forgive himself for his irrational behavior through the practice of self-compassion. He armed himself with tools for thriving at work through the counseling sessions on areas like setting boundaries, prioritization, clarifying roles and responsibilities which were some of the challenges faced at work that contributed to the disengagement, low sense of personal accomplishment and later, severe emotional exhaustion and physical symptoms like the chronic pain experienced. The emotional exhaustion had caused Kai to fall asleep right after work, with just enough energy to have dinner with his family and shower until the next morning.

While off work, Kai has continued to eat healthy and been able to exercise more consistently by going on hikes or long walks, and has also challenged the cognitive distorted thoughts he gets; such as *'it was your fault you lost your job'*. The truth was that his organization was downsizing and two of his other colleagues were also laid off work about a month later. He has been able to let go of some toxic relationships he had, built new connections in his community, and appears to be thriving better.

He feels ready to go back to work as his energy level has been renewed. He is no longer sleep-deprived having reset his sleep-wake biological clock while waiting for another job opportunity. With the help of his therapist, Kai has also had time to re-evaluate his background culture which fosters *'work, work, work harder'* and has committed to creating time for self through the new practice of regular self-renewal.

Angie, who is still off-work for some weeks now, sees her primary care provider quite regularly. She is taking professional courses on improving mental health and wellbeing which she says will help prepare her for going back to work healthier. She continues to be active, walking her dog every day. The length of time it takes to reset from burnout varies and is likely dependent on the severity. A reduction in workforce is one of many consequences of burnout. Angie is also nursing the idea of making a career switch, like Curt.

For Andrew it was different. He simply needed to know what was wrong with him, which sadly he thought was related to toxic workplace and issues bordering on racism and discrimination. He made some work-related changes that helped improve things for him. His leader was understanding and supportive of the need to take needed time off work to reset and recharge. Andrew continues to focus on improving his wellness- resilience bank account, in the event he suffers a short-term stressful situation in his role as an engineer.

THE ROLE OF LIFE COACH[40]

A coach is not a mental health therapist. Coaches could be useful resources for many and while some are certified, others are not. Some focus on specific aspects such as health or career, while others do it all. Life coaching draws upon positive psychological techniques, cognitive-behavioral and solution-focused therapies to help people thrive beyond the workplace, through increased self-awareness, strength-building, and application of the insights generated in moving forward.[39]

During life coaching, the work is done by the individual and not the therapist. The solutions are those that the individual comes up with during sessions and they are held accountable to start making those changes by the coach.

Kai is currently utilizing the services of both a career coach and a therapist to help her stay the course. Some organizations have worker benefits that could help cover the cost of using professionals like career coaches or psychologists. This could be an area worth exploring.

Not everyone needs a career coach or psychologist to recover from burnout; it depends on the severity and personal circumstances. In Curt's case, he switched careers from accounting to the Police Force, hoping to offer compassionate policing drawing on his newly learned mental health skills. Curt took ownership of what he truly wanted out of life and discarded the people-pleasing culture he grew up with whereby he went into accounting field to make his parents happy. He also had to create work boundaries to maintain work-life balance.

Trish, Curt's partner, moved from a strictly on-site full-time work to hybrid work, with a modified schedule that avoided high traffic congestion. Trish is doing well and has not made a career change. Both she and Curt now have more time for their relationship which I understand is going to be consummated sometime soon.

ROLE OF FINANCIAL ADVISORS AND ACCOUNTANTS

I had mentioned earlier that personal culture and its relationship with finances can be a burnout driver,[4,40] for instance, the individual dealing with the consequences of financial errors, or takes on the financial burden of others (family members) requiring that they take on two or more jobs or work longer hours to make ends mee. Another burnout driver that is unrelated to family culture is heavy financial burden for the individual who does not have free healthcare as we do in Canada, or insufficient health insurance to cover the treatment expense of grave medical diagnosis like cancer. I like many others had little knowledge of the role of accountants other than tax purposes, or the actual benefit of having financial advisors until later in life.

Let me share a little of my background as it relates to finances and some of the ills of culture. I had been curious about money management as early as high school days when I first took Economics as a course. I went home and sought dad's audience during which my observation about his spending habit was shared with him. He was basically a philanthropist to a fault. He spent a lot more helping other people and family members than he was earning.

Whenever we went to our hometown, it seemed that an alarm had sounded overnight as I would wake up in the morning to see many people in our sitting areas. They needed help with school fees for their kids, paying their medical bills, and even getting married. Dad had also built the first town hall in my hometown decades ago. To my suggestion that he invested in more productive ventures like transport service he had a good laugh. He reassured me we would be alright.

Dad was kindhearted but he like many had his flaws too, and we won't go there in depth. One of such was that he was a polygamist and that meant many wives and kids, a view informed by the Igbo tradition and culture. As a product of his excesses, it is hard to condemn his ways anyway, or can I?

However, I learned from his mistakes and so had an early start to balancing my earning with spending. I learned firsthand not to allow the culture that drove dad from being someone who had more than enough to living from pay cheque-to-pay cheque. The point here being to consider balancing 'saving for rainy day' with people pleasing and excessive generosity at one's own detriment.

As an immigrant to Canada, I found out that the old financial wisdom that worked well in the previous setting would not serve me fully. That also led me to buy and read books like *The Wealthy Barber* by David Chilton[41] *Never Too Late* by Gaile Vaz-Oxlade.[31] The quest for improvement in every area of one's life is the key to seeking out knowledge, and skills, and their application is even equally vital for change to occur. This is true whether one is an apprentice, or a recent graduate from any professional program. Without the application of theory through practice, that knowledge becomes at best redundant.

In the days when I had a nine-to five job, I was able to file my income tax myself using Tax apps, no problem. My employer took out the taxes before I got my pay cheque so the need for an accountant was not felt. It seemed easy. But as a practicing physician, it's more complicated because one is self-employed and not assigning enough taxes proactively has led many to experience stress during their year-end or after corporation income tax has been filed and reviewed by the government.

As things became more complex, I realized the need for an accountant to assist with income tax filings.

To prevent and manage my financial stress, I enlisted the services of an accountant who in my view, has been a Godsend. If they didn't accommodate some of my administrative inefficiencies, more money would be lost to the system compared with the cost of their accounting services.

Financial advisors suggest that people consider taking out life insurance, making time to create wills and advance care directives, investing in stocks and bonds and real estate. The thing to look out for, from my experience, is a financial advisor who can provide one with a much broader financial picture than what one could themselves. This means being courageous to test drive until one finds the advisor that challenges them to think outside the box. No, I am not a high-risk investor. If it were possible to go to bed with my money under my pillow, I would do that. You ever heard of people who like to be able to hold their, as in be able to see it? I'm one of those, because any investment with the potential to increase my financial gain but equally lose it overnight is a scary thought.

Sometimes I wonder if perception of wealth and family circumstances requiring one start life afresh at age forty has contributed to my rather conservative investment mentality. To me, depending on one's circumstances, it make sense to initially forgo those extras that make life more fun until one has a solid financial base, before taking more risks and also indulging on things that count as wants and not needs. This approach provided me with a mental and financial balance; and created room for travel and other things that help ne recharge and reset the stress-burnout button.

My current financial advisor took a different approach from the others before him. He asked questions that helped me clarify my current and future financial goals. He might not have known this but I felt his style qualified as financial coaching. After a few sessions, I had clarity on my finances. Therefore, I asked him what he would want people to know in order to make better financial decisions. He shared that physicians need advisors who have experience working with other physicians as a starting point. Beyond physicians, the tips he shared with me are useful for just about anyone.

The key areas where he thought that good advisors demonstrate the value of the fees charged are:

- *Getting a sense of people's life priorities and the desired future life. He opined that this aspect gets 'unlocked' only by a joint discussion and the line of inquiry the advisor pursues.*
- *Assisting clients determine their cash flow and aligning it with the current realities and the desired future state. For example, if one desires to have enough retirement savings, it requires some intentionality and money discipline.*
- *The third step requires the building of a financial plan that aligns with the client's goals and circumstances, with input from the client's accountants, ensuring that all decisions made align.*
- *Additionally, there is a need to prioritize investing over debt repayment, with some guidance around investing in the most tax-efficient ways. My take on this, is one of balance and people's comfort level. Generally, I dislike owing. My threshold for debt repayment is quite low; meaning I often focus on reducing my debt, and find ways to balance that out with some level of investment. Again for everyone and their unique circumstances, it will be different.*
- *Ensuring that incapacity and estate plans are in place is important because they are potential sources of subconscious stress and (although he shared a few more tips, let's end on the note that)*
- *Without a clear vision, an overwhelming workload can quickly overcome even the strongest people.*

And since no single financial plan is entirely 'set and forget', semi-annual or annual meetings are considered part of good financial health, as taking one's car for a tune-up or seeing one's primary care provider to enhance good physical health.

PERSONAL AND PROFESSIONAL DEVELOPMENT

As a young girl, although some thought I was 'bossy', I wonder if there were obvious leadership qualities that led to being selected as class prefect in elementary school or dining room prefect in High School. This in some ways suggests that leaders were born to lead, however, that school of thought is balanced with the knowledge of the possibility of training just about anyone who is willing to lead. The problem with 'natural leaders', assuming there was ever such thing, is that without proper training, they are likely to falter and cause unintended harm to others. Nonetheless we must start from somewhere.

Trained or not, when people with the skills and knowledge that can contribute to positive workplace changes do not step up to take on leadership roles, it is a disservice to them and others. How can change happen if we all prefer to play it safe and not take risks? Hence, my suggestion is that people who have volunteered or been appointed to lead seek self-improvement opportunities since they are the best assessor of the hidden gaps they might have. This is being mentioned in this section as a personal strategy for improving self, because of the potential to impact to improve the workplace culture.

Effective Communication skills training, Conflict Management, Mindfulness-Based Stress Reduction Strategies, coaching in the workplace and other resources promoting work-life integration are some areas that leaders may wish to consider availing themselves of for both self-improvement and professional development.

It is that quest for improvement that led me to find continuous learning opportunities such as medical and mental health conferences, personal development workshops on topics like communication skills, managing effective meetings, managing and engaging others, and trauma informed leadership. I am also undergoing training to become a *life coach* because of my desire to support my clients in adopting and maintaining changes that will improve their physical health and mental wellbeing. Since my ultimate goal in life is to improve lives, wherever I go, I make sure I am ready to offer great value.

This also means that there's the realization that with any leadership role I land, there is the possibility of improving lives in meaningful ways, and along with that the risk of facing structural barriers. I've heard it being said that if one must cause trouble, they should consider making good trouble and that doesn't necessarily resonate with me.

I believe that change is possible if we desire it and are ready to find meaningful and effective solutions. Giving up without trying hard to effect change goes against the core of the grain of my fabric.

CHAPTER TEN

RECHARGED AND READY

You are the Chief executive Officer (C.E.O.) of your health, and your life. This position requires taking full stock of where one is at, assessing the presence or absence of burnout, identifying the various stress-burnout drivers, and coming up with holistic strategies that either prevent it or allow for complete recovery. Anything less will be ineffective.

By making the needed change to improve work situations and develop self-efficacy and self-renewal incorporating physical, mental (and spiritual, if so inclined) strategies, one's success at thriving is guaranteed. Reflecting on other personal factors fueling workplace burnout and utilizing a multi-faceted approach for mitigating burnout, the higher the chance that one's healing will last the test of time. These approaches have the additional benefit of building a fatter wellness- resilience bank account, the buffer for dealing with those curveballs that life throws every so often.

Mindfulness offers another tool for checking how one is doing; just like using a thermometer to assess if one had fever. This means that mindfulness could serve as a daily gauge for assessing how one is doing physically, emotionally, behaviourally and otherwise. Sometimes, one could hold self-accountable by asking a trusted co-worker to be a sounding board for calling them out if their actions are not in alignment with their core values. A consistent practice of checking how one is doing and tackling problems early on could help prevent burnout, with a quicker turnaround time for resetting and recharging. The body provides one enough cue that a mental and physical tune up is needed

Indeed, no one organization has it all, and so as humans there will be days when things don't make sense. Finding someone who one trusts at work to play the role of sounding board could be another way of dealing with workplace frustrations. The relationship needs to be one in which there is psychological safety mean while being confident that the individual has your best interest at heart.

As someone who enjoys colorful and tasty meals, getting back to work with a full tank equal having a medley of all the different essential ingredients in the right proportions to make for a healthy worker and psychologically safe workplaces. Some of these ingredients (human and material resources and wellness culture) must be provided by the workplace for the individual to thrive. Remember, it is always a good idea to improve self, increase one's knowledge and skills which are sure to be come in handy, in the event the tough decision needs to be made to jump ship and or, change career course.

Nobody was created to be an island. The richer your work, home, community *'inner circle'* and professional *'connections'*, the better at thriving you will be. There is certainly a role for primary care providers such as a Family doctor or Nurse Practitioner, a counsellor, a financial advisor, an accountant at minimum. The reason is that these individuals have the knowledge and skills to improve one's health and finances than any Google doctor or book can. Some may need spiritual leader, or career coach depending on the circumstances and people's unique needs, there could be a role for dietitian, physiotherapist, occupational therapist or a lawyer. It would be wise to also consider getting life insurance, and a will done, and the consideration for legal input, if one's estate is complex. To do a full scope review and balance own solutions with some professional assistance, will go a long way in 'keeping one's house in order'.

The work of a certified coach goes beyond preparation for job hunting, assisting with applications, to guiding the individual in discovering own solutions for work or home challenges. The role of a coach differs from that of counsellor (mental health therapist) in that the latter offers a deeper-dive into areas that ultimately create room for self-development, self-discovery, and relationship-building, with suggestions or new strategies for thriving wherever people find themselves.

Oftentimes financial strain or the fear of being in need can drive individuals into work longer hours to make ends meet. Investing in a financial advisor and or an accountant to assess financial health could be helpful in guiding savings, investments, and tax implications. For the spiritually inclined, connecting with and confiding in religious leaders or others who share similar beliefs has the potential to keep you grounded and in balance.

Surrounding oneself with authentic friends and supportive family members in a healthy relationship where there is vulnerability, open communication, love for one another and holding each other accountable. At different times and seasons, one might find themselves providing nurture and the roles reversed as seasons change. To not be recharged from time-to-time and to feel drained are signs of a 'not-so-healthy' relationship. Utilizing the practice of mindfulness is one way to evaluate friendships as a way of keeping it healthy and balanced.

Personal Healing Strategies

Adopting a healthy lifestyle:
- Eating healthy diet
- Fitness
- Good sleep hygiene
- Hydration
- Safe alcohol limits
- Limit caffeinated drinks

Adopting new hobbies or pass times that are fulfilling:
- Travel
- Singing
- Play an instrument
- Swimming
- Journaling
- Learn a new language

Create time for the practice of mindfulness and meditation:
- Environmental and body scan reflexive exercises while at work
- Consider setting aside a mental health day as reminder for self care

Investing in Professional development and increasing skill set:
- Acquiring additional skills can be advantageous for promotion and, in the case of an unhealthy work environment, can broaden a worker's perspective, equipping them with relevant and valuable capabilities

Healing With Others

- **Social networking with friends, family and co-workers**
- **Drawing on higher powers (spirituality):**
  - Seeking guidance or prayers from pastors, priests, chaplains, Imams, and other religious leaders
- **Volunteering**

Work Related Strategies

- Boundary-setting
- Prioritization
- Avoid excessive multi-tasking
- Delegate
- Ask for help early
- Adopt healthy work practices
- Build work coalitions
- Utilize human resource department staff for work-related issues around work culture
- Participate in wellness initiatives at work

Professional Care

- Primary care provider
- Psychologist
- Career coach
- Accountant & Financial Advisor

Figure 6: Overall Holistic strategies for mitigating burnout

OTHER SELF MAINTENANCE APPROACHES

Listening to materials that build one up – podcasts, talks, trainings, sessions, books are a few ideas for learning and growing. Figure 6 is an attempt at putting it all together for the worker, a full scope care for thriving in the workplace.

REFLECTION QUESTIONS

1. Who is in your inner circle now, could be one to three individuals? Draw and write down their names and their roles.
2. Are there names of people you have a relationship with, that you have been having misgivings about? Did you write down the name of any of the individuals you have misgivings about in the inner circle? If so, please cross out their names for now. It's okay to not have three names for example. The list grows when mutual trust, respect and common values are the guiding principles. There can be other core values that matter to you so please create your list based on your own values.

In the circle external to the inner circle you drew above, please add another circle encompassing the inner one. Please add one or more individuals for their potential professional role in your current situation? Can you commit to reaching out to them in the next week or two now that you have identified a gap and a need to close that gap?

ACTION PLAN

Remember that what you cannot measure, you cannot assess. Please list areas you need to work on to improve your overall health and mental wellbeing. Write down as many as you can. Give specific examples of the goals for each domain. For example, boundary-setting, healthy diet, exercise, rest, and making healthy social connections. Which of these are your top three to five?

Please note that each change or specific area you are committing to requires spending a minimum of three to four weeks before embarking on the next another goal.

Using the **'SMART'** Acronym, write these down

Specific: This is the goal you wish to achieve
Measurable: How will you evaluate if you have made progress
Achievable: Is the goal you have set something that can be done
Realistic: How realistic is the goal you set for yourself? If it isn't realistic, revisit the goal again
Timeline: In what timeframe do you hope to achieve your new goal? Make sure it is reasonable

Of the list you created, which areas need revision or modification? Can you start with one priority area by this weekend or next Monday? What is holding you back? What can you do to mitigate the barrier?

When you hit a roadblock preventing you from committing to making change(s):

Appreciate that life happens and sometimes even with the best intent, delays can arise. However, no excuse is good enough long term for not committing to change. If you do have to defer making a change, please write down how much time you are giving yourself and then set a reminder on your phone's or other calendar to revisit the commitment to change action plan.

When you hit roadblock having begun to make changes:

Please write down the changes that you have made over the last month and what you were able to achieve at the end of the three- to-four-week period. Review these and continue with the new lifestyle to keep you going like a well-oiled machine. Well done!!

You are worth every investment and effort you make to keep healthy. I have been impressed a few times by some seniors whose paths I came across in the last couple of decades. This is because at eighty or ninety plus years, I admire that they have managed to remain quite active and appear to be enjoying life to the full.

CONCLUSION

As I said earlier, no situation ever improved from doing nothing.

First, we identified the elements of burnout as emotional exhaustion, depersonalization in which one is likely to be cynical and detached from one's work, and lack of professional fulfillment.

We also evaluated the role of culture as a burnout driver; system and organizational culture have a higher propensity in driving burnout in workers. The downside to negative culture is a high work turnover, absenteeism, sickness-presenteeism and burnout, to name a few.

Although burnout is work-related, there are personal traits and characteristics that increase the chance of burnout in people. For instance, people's family background and culture which also includes parental and societal expectations, and personal traits like people-pleasing or workaholic are contributors in exacerbating burnout.

The ability to assess burnout drivers in self in a holistic manner and identify strategies that help mitigate it will go a long way in the healing journey and ability to thrive in the workplace longer. An approach that combines physical, mental, social, and spiritual domains are likely to produce better results than narrow focused ones. Remember these allow one to improve their wellness-resilience bank account and encouraged self-compassion and kindness. For without self-love, it can be rather challenging to offer to others what one does not have to give to self. The practice of mindfulness can be helpful in keeping things in perspective. Additionally, when nothing seems to be helping, consider booking an appointment with your family doctor to rule out other potential causes of extreme fatigue.

There are many ways to assess readiness to change and one model that we were taught during our residency training was the Proschaka and DiClemente's Cycle of Change. The change cycle consists of the pre-contemplative, contemplative, preparation, action, maintenance and relapse which are useful in assessing a client or patient's readiness to make changes. For example, if one is at the pre-contemplative phase, the chance of making any change is a lot more challenging, even with coaching. The advantage of having counseling or health coaching is that it could be useful in moving the individual to the next phase of the change cycle, for example, contemplative to preparation. It would be to no one's advantage to stick one's gun when a change is necessary because of its ability to impact the individual's health and wellbeing.

Steve Covey talked about commitment to change through the idea of an *upward spiral*. The principle and process of renewal occurs through growth and change, with a continuous practice of improvement taking place in a spiral-upwards fashion[42].

For instance, assuming an individual wished to stop the habit of taking work home. The process starts with identifying the issue, in this case work-life imbalance and decides to stop the habit, this constitutes the *'learn'*, setting a date to effect the change is the *'commit'*, and when the individual starts to implement boundary-setting; the *'do'*. There remains a need to invest in a maintenance culture or phase to ensure that one thrives. This is the phase where the individual might wish to consider injecting new strategies or adapting the steps being taken to ensure they do not get bored or tired from monotony.

What commitment are you willing to make to heal from burnout, or other physical and mental health issues? Any change made to tackle burnout will likely help improve one's holistic health because of the multi-faceted approach suggested in this book. Remember the saying that Rome was not built in a day? Please remember to be kind and compassionate to self, knowing that the current position one is at did not happen overnight. That is, it will take some time to see lasting, so please be patient.

For instance, if the last time you wore a size twelve dress or outfit was four years ago and you are now a size sixteen, it is important to slowly work one's way down to size fourteen first before size twelve. To rush the process means there will likely be a higher chance of experiencing hiccups or setbacks. Setbacks are allowed only momentarily, before getting back on track.

Plan to involve a professional — career coach, spiritual mentor, family physician, therapist, financial advisor— and a circle of trusted friends and family members. They keep you accountable and provide a broader perspective.

Nothing will give me more joy than hearing your stories of not just overcoming burnout in a positive manner, but also of thriving better in the workplace and home setting. I'm rooting for you and your improved wellness states.

I can be reached via the following means:

Instagram: dr.florence.obianyor
FaceBook: Dr.Flo.net
Email: drobianyor@gmail.com

APPENDIX

Figure 1: Car-burnout analogy
Figure 2: Diagram of Culture and its relationship to burnout
Figure 3: brain image
Figure 4: Work-related Healing strategies
Figure 5: Diagram of personal strategies
Figure 6: Overall Holistic strategies for mitigating burnout
Figure 7: This diagram is specific to Family Physicians and the challenges they face in clinical practice and highlights solutions to those specific areas as well.

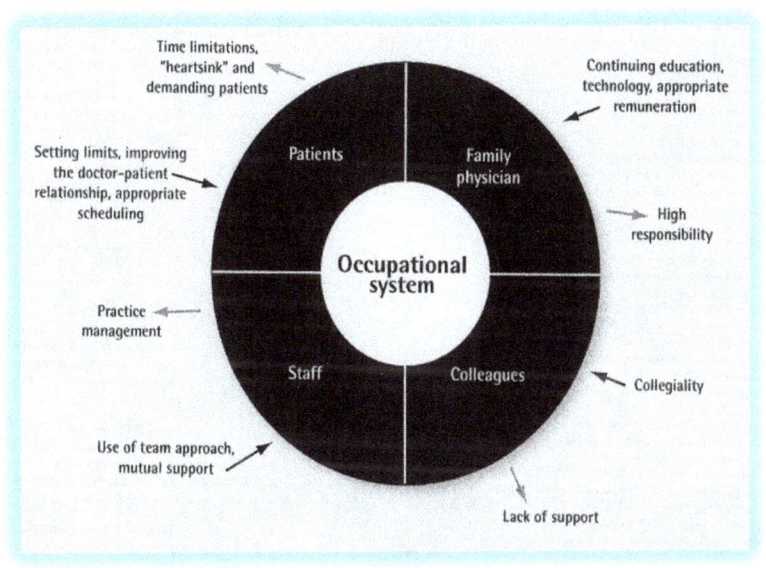

Figure 7: The occupational system: Outward arrows indicate negative inputs (stresses) that diminish the system and inward arrows indicate positive inputs (strategies) that augment the system. By Dr. Lee and colleagues (2008)

REFERENCES

1. Lawrence JA, Davis BA, Corbette T, Hill EV, Williams DR, Reede JY. Racial/Ethnic Differences in Burnout: a Systematic Review. J Racial Ethn Health Disparities. 2022 Feb;9(1):257-269. doi: 10.1007/s40615-020-00950-0. Epub 2021 Jan 11. PMID: 33428158; PMCID: PMC7799165.
2. Thomas, N. K. (2004). Resident burnout. JAMA, 292(23), 2880-2889
3. World Health Organization. Definition of Burnout. Retrieved from: https://www.who.int/news/item/28-05-2019-burn-out-an-occupational-phenomenon-international-classification-of-diseases. Accessed September 26,2023
4. Lee, F. J., Brown, J. B., & Stewart, M. (2009). Exploring family physician stress: Helpful strategies. Canadian Family Physician, 55(3), 288-289.e6
5. Ratanawongsa, N., Roter, D., Beach, M. C., Laird, S. L., Larson, S. M., Carson, K. A., et al. (2008). Physician burnout and patient-physician communication during primary care encounters. Journal of General Internal Medicine, 23(10), 1581-1588.
6. Soler, J. K., Yaman, H., Esteva, M., Dobbs, F., Asenova, R. S., Katic, M., et al. (2008). Burnout in european family doctors: The EGPRN study. Family Practice, 25(4), 245-265.
7. CMA 2021 National Physician Health Survey. Available https://www.cma.ca/sites/default/files/2022-08/
8. Nurses: Working harder, more hours amid increased labour shortage - Statistics Canada. Accessed December 1, 2023, from https://www.statcan.gc.ca/o1/en/plus/4165-nurses-working-harder-more-hours-amid-increased-labour-shortage
9. Tara Haelle, 2020; Your surge capacity is depleted. It's why you feel awful. Our Brains Struggle to Process This Much Stress | Elemental (medium.com) Accessed August 17,2023.

10. Kim, H., Shin, K., & Hwang, J. (2023). Too much may be a bad thing: the difference between challenge and hindrance job demands. Current psychology (New Brunswick, N.J.), 1–13.
11. Yerkes, R. M., & Dodson, J. D. (1908). The Relation of Strength of Stimulus to Rapidity of Habit-Formation. Journal of Comparative Neurology and Psychology, 18, 459-482. http://dx.doi.org/10.1002/cne.920180503.
12. Lepnurm, R., Dobson, R., Backman, A., & Keegan, D. (2007). Factors associated with career satisfaction among general practitioners in Canada. Canadian Journal of Rural Medicine, 12(4), 217-230.
13. Bréne Brown (2021, 6)Atlas of the Heart: Mapping Meaningful Connection and the Language of Human Experience. Random House Publishing Group
14. Li-Sauerwine S, Rebillot K, Melamed M, Addo N, Lin M. A 2-Question Summative Score Correlates with the Maslach Burnout Inventory. West J Emerg Med. 2020 Apr 21;21(3):610-617. doi: 10.5811/westjem.2020.2.45139. PMID: 32421508; PMCID: PMC7234685.
15. West CP, Dyrbye LN, Shanafelt TD. Physician burnout: contributors, consequences and solutions. J Intern Med. 2018 Jun;283(6):516-529. doi: 10.1111/joim.12752. Epub 2018 Mar 24. PMID: 29505159.
16. Krasner, M. S., Epstein, R. M., Beckman, H., Suchman, A. L., Chapman, B., Mooney, C. J., et al. (2009). Association of an educational program in mindful communication with burnout, empathy, and attitudes among primary care physicians. JAMA, 302(12), 1284-1293.
17. Twellaar, M., Winants, Y., & Houkes, I. (2008). How healthy are dutch general practitioners? self-reported (mental) health among dutch general practitioners. European Journal of General Practice, 14(1), 4-9.
18. Mate, Gabor (2004) When the Body Says No: The Hidden Cost of Stress. Vintage Canada
19. Culture Definition & Meaning - Merriam-Webster. Accessed October 17, 2023
20. Martin M. Physician Well-Being: Physician Burnout. FP Essent. 2018 Aug;471:11-15. PMID: 30107104.

21. Stordeur S, Vandenberghe C, D'hoore W. Prédicteurs de l'épuisement professionnel des infirmières: une étude dans un hôpital universitaire [Predictors of nurses' professional burnout: a study in a university hospital]. Rech Soins Infirm. 1999 Dec;(59):57-67. French. PMID: 12037845.
22. Arnsten AFT, Shanafelt T. Physician Distress and Burnout: The Neurobiological Perspective. Mayo Clin Proc. 2021 Mar;96(3):763-769. doi: 10.1016/j.mayocp.2020.12.027. PMID: 33673923; PMCID: PMC7944649
23. Romani M, Ashkar K. Burnout among physicians. Libyan J Med. 2014 Feb 17;9(1):23556. doi: 10.3402/ljm.v9.23556. PMID: 24560380; PMCID: PMC3929077.
24. Joiner Jr. T.E., Kimberly A. Van Orden, Tracy K. Witte, Edward A. Selby, Jessica D. Ribeiro, and Robyn Lewis, M. David Rudd. Journal of Abnormal Psychology 2009, Vol. 118, No. 3, 634–646
25. Salvagioni DAJ, Melanda FN, Mesas AE, González AD, Gabani FL, Andrade SM. Physical, psychological and occupational consequences of job burnout: A systematic review of prospective studies. PLoS One. 2017 Oct 4;12(10):e0185781. doi: 10.1371/journal.pone.0185781. PMID: 28977041; PMCID: PMC5627926.
26. Lemaire,W. J.B and Ghali, W. A. (2009). Physician wellness: A missing quality indicator. Lancet, 374(9702), 1714-1721.
27. Shanafelt, T. D., & Noseworthy, J. H. (2017). Executive Leadership and Physician Well-being: Nine Organizational Strategies to Promote Engagement and Reduce Burnout. Mayo Clinic proceedings, 92(1), 129–146. https://doi.org/10.1016/j.mayocp.2016.10.004
28. Maddeus M. The Resilience Bank Account: Skills for Optimal Performance. Ann Thorac Surg. 2020 Jan;109(1):18-25. doi: 10.1016/j.athoracsur.2019.07.063. Epub 2019 Sep 10. PMID: 31518588.
29. Davis, Martha, Elizabeth R. Eshelman, and Matthew McKay. 2008. The Relaxation & Stress Reduction Workbook. N.p.: New Harbinger Publications (Pg 221-225, 297-308)
30. Davich, Victor N. 1998. The Best Guide to Meditation: This is the Perfect Book If You Want to Reduce Stress, If You Already Meditate But Want to Learn New Techniques, Or If You're Just Curious About How it Works. N.p.: St. Martin's Publishing Group.

31. Vaz-Oxlade, G (2010): Never too Late-Take Control of Your Retirement and Your Life. Collins.
32. Peterkin, Allan. (2008Pg26-33, 41-54,) . Staying Human During Residency Training: How to Survive and Thrive After Medical School. N.p.: University of Toronto Press.
33. Canada's Food Guide (2019) Retrieved from : https://food-guide.canada.ca/en/. Accessed October 5th,2023.
34. Siler, Brooke. 2000. The Pilates Body: The Ultimate At-Home Guide to Strengthening, Lengthening and Toning Your Body-Without Machines. N.p.: Harmony/Rodale
35. DASH DIET. Retrieved from: https://www.mayoclinic.org/healthy-lifestyle/nutrition-and-healthy-eating/in-depth/dash-diet/art-20048456 Accessed October 19, 2023.
36. Cancer Screening.Retrieved from: https://screeningforlife.ca/ Accessed OCtober 19, 2023
37. Benson, J., & Magraith, K. (2005). Compassion fatigue and burnout: the role of Balint groups. Australian family physician, 34(6), 497–498.
38. Jensen, P. M., Trollope-Kumar, K., Waters, H., & Everson, J. (2008). Building physician resilience. Canadian family physician Medecin de famille canadien, 54(5), 722–729.
39. Southwick, S.M.,Bonanno, G.A.,,. Masten, A.S.,Panter-Brick,C. & Yehuda,R. (2014). Resilience definitions, theory, and challenges: interdisciplinary perspectives, European Journal of Psychotraumatology, 5:1, DOI: 10.3402/ejpt.v5.25338
40. Askin,W.J. Coaching for physicians: building more resilient doctors. Can Fam Physician. 2008 Oct;54(10):1399-400. PMID: 18854466; PMCID: PMC2567251.
41. Chilton, D. (1989).The Wealthy Barber. The Common Sense Guide To Financial Planning. Stoddart Publishing Co. Limited.
42. Covey, Stephen R. (2013, 317-318). The 7 Habits of Highly Effective People: Powerful Lessons in Personal Change. N.p.: Simon & Schuster

GLOSSARY OF TERMS

Burnout

Defined as a syndrome arising from chronic stress that has not been successfully managed that consists of three components:
- *Feelings of energy depletion or exhaustion;*
- *Increased mental distance from one's job, or feelings of negativism or cynicism related to one's job; and*
- *Reduced professional efficacy.'*

Culture

Culture is defined as *'the customary beliefs, social forms, and material traits of a racial, religious, or social group.'*

HR

Human resources

LEADS Framework

LEADS framework stands for *Lead Self, Engage Others, Achieve Results, Develop Coalitions and System Transformation*

Mindfulness

Mindfulness includes:
- *Body scan: in which you notice bodily sensations and the cognitive and emotional reactions associated with those sensations without an attempt to change the sensations;*
- *Sitting meditation: involves silent meditation in a seated position that brings awareness to thoughts, feelings, and sensations experienced in the moment;*
- *Walking meditation: brings awareness to the experience of slow, deliberate, and attentive walking; and*
- *Mindful movement: this includes yoga-type exercises done in a way that allows the exploration of the sensory, emotional, and cognitive aspects of the experience.*

OQCE

OQCE stands for *'over qualification without Canadian experience'*

Resilience

Resilience can be looked at from three perspectives, *i) personalization in which individuals believe they are the problem, ii) permanence arising from cognitive distortions that suggest that the challenging situation is here to stay creating more stress and anxiety, and lastly iii) pervasiveness which contributes to the feeling of despair and despondency where hope becomes quite blurry and 'nothing good is left'*

Sickness-Presenteesim

Sickness-Presenteeism is a situation whereby minor health problems are ignored despite the awareness that taking sick leave is necessary.

Surge Capacity

Surge capacity is defined as the physical and mental adaptive systems that individuals draw upon for short term survival of stressful situations.

Trauma

Individual trauma results from an event, series of events, or set of circumstances that is experienced by an individual as physically or emotionally harmful or life threatening and that has lasting adverse effects on the individual's functioning and mental, physical, social, emotional, or spiritual well-being.

Trauma-informed

Trauma-informed care is an approach that recognizes and responds to the impact of trauma by creating a safe environment, fostering trust, and addressing individuals' unique needs to promote healing and prevent re-traumatization.

Work COLA

Work COLA stands for a work *'culture of a lack of authenticity'*

ABOUT THE AUTHOR

Dr. Florence Obianyor has been a physician for over two decades. Since 2011, she has combined primary care with seniors care and mental health and wellbeing, prioritizing client-centered therapy, having moved to Canada.

Now in a pivotal career phase, she is actively contributing to leadership and systemic improvements within her sphere of influence.

Besides writing, her hobbies are global travel, entertaining and hiking.

ABOUT THE BOOK

Have you ever felt like you're running on empty, with nothing left to give to your job, your family, or even yourself? Then join the conversation with someone who's been there. As a seasoned Family Physician and Generalist in Mental Health, Dr. Florence Obianyor (aka Dr. Flo) has seen firsthand how burnout can sneak up on the most dedicated professionals in many industries. Her mission is to raise awareness, empower individuals to reclaim their physical and mental well-being, and foster a thriving work life.

In this book, Dr. Flo explores the different cultural, societal, organizational and personal drivers of burnout, and provides a holistic burnout recovery approach that helps address the root problem. She invites you into her personal space as she shares her experiences and those of her clients who have suffered from burnout. She also shares self-reflective exercises and personal resources to help you combat the burnout beast and return to work with a full tank of energy and enthusiasm.

Join her to take charge of your well-being and make rewarding lifestyle changes so you can start thriving rather than surviving.

www.ingramcontent.com/pod-product-compliance
Lightning Source LLC
Chambersburg PA
CBHW051548020426
42333CB00016B/2154